PRAISE FOR *RESILIENCE*

"A must-read book for anyone diagnosed with cancer or living with someone diagnosed with cancer. This book captures the journey of how dealing with disease affects the psyche. Wener relates her quest to explore alternative ways of dealing with her illnesses, while continuing to use the benefits of traditional medicine. She tells her story with humility and transparency. Her story is a model of resilience, courage, and honesty.

DIANE GUERRERA, *breast cancer survivor and founder of the CURE Foundation*

"Through this extraordinary window into her thoughts, her fears, her defeats, and her triumphs, we come to understand Susan Wener not simply as a "case" but as a whole person. As a physician, this book gives me the opportunity to think about how I can do more for my patients by being a better listener and by trying harder to understand them as individuals rather than cases. As someone responsible for the education of students and residents, *Resilience* has given me food for thought about how we can better prepare the next generation of physicians."

DAVID EIDELMAN, MD, CM, *Dean, Faculty of Medicine, McGill University*

"If the word resilience had a face, it would have to be Susan Wener's. She is the proof that physical fragility, emotional distress, and fear can be overcome. Everyone, sick or healthy, will benefit from learning Susan's lessons about life, humility, hope, perseverance, and love."

LISE WATIER, *founder, Lise Watier Cosmetics*

"At some point in our life, everyone will face challenges. The quality of our lives will depend on how well we cope during these difficult times. Susan shares her story and the way she and her family lived through this highly emotional and painful period. It is a remarkable story of Susan's strength. Her love for her family, compassion for others in need, and wisdom continued to grow in spite of her pain. Rather than scars, Susan gained a radiant, beautiful spirit that nourishes all of us fortunate enough to spend time with her. I am grateful to Susan for the book she wrote and her spirit that gives me hope."

RUBIN BECKER MD, FRCPC

"Insightful, moving, and easy-to-read, this story takes the reader through the challenges, the setbacks, the fears, and the different strategies to cope with cancer. It offers a message of hope, perseverance, and optimism."

DR. ANDRE LISBONA, MD, FRCPC

"As a general internist and palliative medicine specialist, I am very interested in doctor-patient communication. *Resilience* teaches us so much about how patients want to be communicated with and how important it is to listen to them. I hope that this book serves as a foundation for reflection and change for anyone journeying through a serious illness. If you encounter adversity, think back to the principles that Susan teaches us: believe in and love yourself, talk with and include your family in your decision-making process, keep a good team, and heal by helping others."

GIL KIMEL, MD, MSC, FRCPC

"To know Susan Wener is to get a glimpse of the inner peace that is the goal of every guru, priest, and New Age life coach. This story of the journey that got her where she is today is equal parts gripping, terrifying, and unbearably sad on the one hand and courageous, instructive, and inspiring on the other. No one would ever choose to follow in her footsteps, but her travelogue is a tool kit for building structures of hope, optimism, and triumph in the neighborhood of disease, suffering, and death."

MICHAEL WALKER, PHD

"A 'must read' for everyone. I loved the book and read it in two sittings with a box of Kleenex. Some of the tears were shed for her deep suffering but many were also shed in joy for her courage, strength, and triumphs!"

GORDON BYRN, *chairman, Carlyle Gordon Limited*

"Susan Wener's poignant description of her battle with colon cancer provides insights into the challenges that face every patient dealing with a life-altering illness. The book also offers an excellent overview of how both traditional Western medicine and complementary/alternative medicine can be beneficial to whole person care. As a result of her many emotional and physical ups and downs, Susan has dedicated her professional career to understanding the importance of a healthy balance between body and mind."

STEPHEN H. CARSON MD, *pediatrician and pediatric pulmonologist*

RESILIENCE

a story *of* courage and triumph
in the face of recurrent cancer

_____

SUSAN WENER

resilience

FIGURE 1 PUBLISHING *Vancouver*

Cataloguing data available from Library and Archives Canada
ISBN 978-1-927958-02-5 (pbk.)
ISBN 978-1-927958-03-2 (ebook)

First edit by David Smajovits
Editing by Shirarose Wilensky
Cover design by Peter Cocking
Text design by Jennifer Griffiths
Cover photograph by © Heather Hryciw/Corbis
Printed and bound in Canada by Friesens
Distributed in the U.S. by Publishers Group West

Figure 1 Publishing Inc.
Vancouver BC Canada
www.figure1pub.com

To the doctors who literally saved my body

To my husband and daughters, who saved my soul

And to Resilience, without which I never

would have made it at all

. . .

CONTENTS

ACKNOWLEDGMENTS

FIRST AND FOREMOST is my husband. He is my life partner and best friend. The strength and devotion he has shown me are beyond anything I might have imagined when I took my wedding vows over forty years ago. He took my hand and to this day has never let go. Please know, Jonathan, that you really are "the wind beneath my wings."

My three beautiful daughters, Jacqueline, Kassy, and Ali, gave me the reason to keep on living. They were so young when I was first diagnosed with cancer. There was still so much to teach them, and I knew that I had to do whatever was necessary to give me more time to mentor them. They surprise me daily with their strength, vitality, and wisdom. They have become my biggest teachers.

I would like to thank my late father, Julius Hanek, whose unconditional love was a constant throughout my adult life. Although you are no longer here with me physically, Daddy, you are never far from my heart.

As for my mother, Miriam Hanek, your audacity and determination cannot be rivaled. The strength you exhibit in pushing forward and crushing any obstacle that may come your way is remarkable. You remind me daily to get my needs met.

I am truly blessed to have two sisters, one by birth and another by choice. To my sister, Linda Birks, I am so grateful to have learned so much from you. You love deeply and give your all to those lucky enough to know you. Diane Potter, you have been there for me when I needed you, whether at four in the morning or four in the afternoon. Thank you for allowing me to lean on you and for never making me feel as though I was a burden. I am honored to have you in my life.

To my brother, Stephen Hanek, know that what you have accomplished is proof that anything is possible!

To all of my extended family, thank you. You gave me the space I needed for my head and the food I needed for my heart.

Special thanks go to Elizabeth (Beth) Legaspi for your continuous love and devotion. No task has ever been too much for you. You have always treated me as though I was a sacred being, and you were always ready to cancel any personal plans should I have needed you. Beth, you are my family, and I love you!

I am one of those lucky people who have been blessed with amazing friends. All of you have supported me in so many ways, loving me when I needed it most and pushing me when I sometimes wanted it least. I am eternally grateful for your friendship. You have taught me that friendship is a gift and a blessing. Know that it is one I cherish deeply.

I would be remiss not to mention one friend in particular. Linda Carson has been by my side for more than fifty years. When we are together, I sometimes still feel as I did when we were little girls, giggling and sharing secrets. I trust you with my life. You love and protect me with the fierceness of a lioness. What a gift it has been to know that a simple phone call is all it takes to have you fly thousands of miles to be with me, just because. You are my heart, and I love you.

I would like to thank David Smajovits, my first editor. You believed in this book right from the start. Thank you for helping me keep one foot ahead of the other and showing me how to "put the lung I may have been missing in my chest back into the book." I would like to thank Shirarose Wilensky, my editor, for her expertise and for pushing me to fill in all the gaps to make the book rich and full. You are a delight to work with.

I would like to thank Dr. Stephen Carson, who showed me how this story contained life lessons so important for each and every one of us.

I would also like to thank Sheila Kussner for founding Hope & Cope. Sheila created a legacy by dedicating her life to helping enrich the lives of those dealing with cancer.

And I would like to thank Nancy Hamilton, who founded the Natural Health Consultants Institute in 1991. The institute helped open my eyes to the world of alternative medicine. It propelled me to continue learning how to get the very best out of both traditional and nontraditional forms of medicine.

Thanks go to Linda Berthiaume, my homeopathic physician, not only for her expertise but for her friendship. You continue to provide me with some very important tools, thus enabling me to live "my very best life."

I would like to thank Shelly Blackwood. You and your team of caregivers kept me safe during a very vulnerable period in my life. Your ability to care for me both physically and emotionally is something I will never forget!

It is difficult to know what to say to a medical team that helped save my life. "Thank you" hardly seems adequate.

To my colorectal surgeon, Dr. Carol-Ann Vasilevsky, thank you for always being there for me. You are not only an incredibly skilled surgeon but a warm, kind, and compassionate woman who took the time to treat not just the illness but also the person.

Thanks go to my medical oncologist, Dr. Alexander Zukiwski. No matter how busy you were, you took whatever time was needed to answer all my questions and offer reassurance. I will never forget how you went above and beyond what might be considered "standard of care."

To Dr. Max Palayew and Dr. André Lisbona, know that your sheer humanity warms my heart. You remind me that compassion can still thrive in a busy hospital setting.

To Dr. Nathan Sheiner, my thoracic surgeon, thank you for giving me the opportunity to watch my family grow up!

To my dear friend Dr. Rubin Becker, thank you. I have probably disturbed more of your sleeps than I would like to admit. You treat your patients with gentleness and sensitivity. You remind your students that helping those who are ill is much more complex than simply treating a malady. You give me hope for the future of medicine, a future where doctors are not afraid to care.

Thanks goes to Dr. Walter Gotlieb, surgical gynecologic oncologist working at the Jewish General Hospital in Montreal. I am honored to have the opportunity to collaborate with you and your team as equals on the gynecology oncology tumor board. I continue to learn and grow because of your mentorship.

I would like the thank Dr. Michael Camilleri, head of gastroenterology at the Mayo Clinic. Your investigative measures ended more than fifteen years of suffering.

Finally, I would like to thank my grandchildren. The dream of having you in my life was something I used to pray for. The thrill of having that dream actualized takes my breath away. Just thinking about you makes my spirit soar. You fill me with sweet joy and wonder, always reminding me of the sacredness, preciousness, and magic of life.

(*foreword*)

THE POWER
OF WORDS

POWERFUL BOOKS CAN change people's lives forever. This inspiring book has certainly done that for me. I read Susan Wener's story in one sitting. I was awed by the straightforward and insightful account of her experience with cancer. She generously provides valuable lessons and describes complementary elements that came her way when the curveball of cancer came into her life.

I met Susan Wener in 2012, when we both served as board members for Hope & Cope. Based at the Jewish General Hospital in Montreal, Quebec, Hope & Cope is a successful organization, run by volunteers and professionals, that supports individuals affected by cancer. Although we had not officially met before that, I had noticed Susan at various cancer-related functions. I was struck by the seemingly paradoxical combination of strong and warm energy that she exuded. The way Susan held herself and spoke publicly showed an exquisite mixture of intelligence, sensitivity, and strength. I could not help but be impressed by how she and her husband, Jonathan Wener, often sat at meetings, side by side like pillars of mutual love, compassion, and determination. I was intrigued by how these strengths might have come about until Susan informed me in passing that she was writing a book about her experience with cancer. She wondered if I could take a look at it.

In the course of my career, as a nurse, a clinical researcher, and a university professor, I have been privileged to witness many personal accounts of people's experience with serious illnesses such as cancer. I remain deeply committed to researching how health professionals can best support and empower individuals and families who are dealing with such challenges. I am particularly impressed by Susan's integrative perspective. Beyond her own journey, Susan has become a recognized expert in supportive approaches that complement traditional forms of cancer treatment. She shows incredible resilience as a person and inspires us to recognize that we must all be open to various means to enhance our well-being. She reminds us to remain hopeful, connected, and proactive—even more so in times of hardship.

I am most honored to be writing this foreword, as I can be unabashedly enthusiastic! Susan has revealed her heart and journey conscientiously and fully. This book is a significant contribution to the healing community and to patients and families who are touched by cancer. Much can be learned from reading this fine exploration of the human spirit.

I am grateful to Susan for her generous sharing of knowledge, experience, and learning with us all.

CARMEN G. LOISELLE, N, PHD
Associate Professor, Faculty of Medicine, McGill University
Christine and Hershel Victor/Hope & Cope Chair in
Psychosocial Oncology
Senior Investigator, Jewish General Hospital
Montreal, February 15, 2013

RESILIENCE

(*prologue*)

RESILIENCE UNCOVERED

THERE IS NO textbook written about how to keep it together when our world is falling apart. Yet for all the curveballs life throws at us, there should be libraries filled with books teaching us how to duck so that we don't get knocked out.

This is a story about transformation and personal growth. Although pain and suffering appear to be the vehicles through which the transformation occurred, the heart of the story lies in the choices we make as a result of what happens to us, rather than in the details of what happens to us.

Few of us know for certain what our futures hold. When we are young, we have a naive feeling of invincibility. We believe that everything is possible, and our destiny holds within itself the quality of magic. As youths, the concept of time has little meaning. If anything, we feel as though time stands still, and we become impatient with its pace. As we age, we realize how quickly time moves and wish we could slow it down. We often try to bargain just to get a little bit more of it.

But what would happen if we got sick? What if we were diagnosed with a life-threatening illness? What if there was no guarantee that we would be alive six months or a year from now? What would the concept of time mean to us then? When we fall ill, the idea of time takes on a whole new meaning. Every second becomes increasingly precious, and the thought of any of it being taken away leaves us frightened and breathless. So many questions race through our minds. What will happen to my family if I die? Who will raise my kids? Will I become a burden to the ones I love most? Will I suffer? Initially, everyone rallies around and support is high. But what about afterwards? What happens if the illness doesn't just go away? What happens when life returns to normal for everyone except for you? How do you simply get on with it? These are some of the issues that I will discuss in the chapters ahead.

When we become sick, we desperately try to find our footing. We look everywhere we can for guidance. Doctors become our allies, and we hunt for tools and strategies to help us make it through. I don't know why some people appear to have a greater capacity to cope than others. Perhaps they are the ones who become our beacons of hope and our inspiration. If they can make it, then we might be able to as well! In this book, I will share some of the tools and strategies I used to help me navigate my way toward health and well-being.

My journey led me on an accelerated path of learning. It forced me to go back to school and helped me to acquire the skills I desperately needed to survive. With the knowledge I gained, I opened up a private practice to help those who are suffering find meaning and joy in their lives, irrespective of circumstance. This story is told from two perspectives: from that of a patient as well as that of a therapist.

Only once I finished writing this book did I realize how long and how deeply I had suffered. Had anyone told me that I would have to deal with physical, mental, and emotional pain for more than thirty years, I would have told them to count me out. No sane person would intentionally sign up for a life like that. Yet in the midst of all I suffered, what awed me most was the fact that I never lost, at least not for very long, my capacity to feel the joy, the beauty, and the sacredness of life. I discovered within myself an internal resilience that I had never recognized before. My experiences led me to understand that my ability to keep bouncing back was instrumental in keeping me alive. It is my hope that from reading this book you will discover, as I did, your own potential and capacity for resilience.

_____

· *resilience* ·

MERRIAM-WEBSTER'S COLLEGIATE DICTIONARY defines resilience as "an ability to recover from or adjust easily to misfortune or change." I am not sure about the easy adjustment part, but the ability to adapt to difficult times often helps us live richer and more productive lives, even when dealing with the unexpected. We are far more capable than any of us might have ever imagined. It is incredible how we somehow seem to find a strength that we never knew existed when confronted with circumstances not of our choosing. Hope, faith, and the belief in possibility have been and are key in helping me keep my head above water.

_____

An anonymous author once wrote: "Everything was once and for a time a dream. The tree lies in the acorn. The bird waits in the egg. The butterfly becomes in the cocoon. Dreams are the seedlings of reality."

I invite you to dare to dream with me, so that you too may open yourself up to the endless possibilities that exist for all of us. For the essence of life, after all, lies not in what is broken but in what we can create.

(1)

BEGINNING AT
THE BEGINNING

I WAS BORN IN 1953, the youngest of three, with a sister named Linda and a brother named Stephen. There were such clear differences between the three of us that it was hard to imagine we came from the same parents. My mother worked hard to keep our family life in order. The house was her domain. She had total responsibility for looking after us. She made sure we were fed, clean, and well behaved. Any free time she had, she devoted to us. She told me I was the easiest of her children. I was completely content on my own, playing for hours in my playpen with anything that was given to me. Because of my contented nature, I never even noticed that my mother spent most of her time addressing the needs of my brother and sister. It seemed that I was born with a happy disposition. Even to this day, there is a sign over my fridge that reads "Don't Bother Me, I Am Living Happily Ever After."

Education was very important to my parents, and they encouraged us to work hard in school. But growing up, I used to spend a lot of my time daydreaming instead of studying. It drove my sister, with whom I shared a bedroom, crazy. It was beyond her how I could sit for hours at my desk with my drawer open, imagining all the things I could fill it with one day. She was the neat and serious one who spent all of her time studying. I was the sloppy, happy-go-lucky one who preferred playing outside and skipping rope. It is no wonder that she drew an invisible line in our room that I was not permitted to cross! I was her antithesis.

My brother was the wild one. There was something inside him that was restless. Adventure was always on his horizon. He was fun. He was exciting. Only eighteen months older than me, he was my playmate and my hero. As the wild one, he got into trouble all the time. I used to sit and weep when he was punished or scolded, feeling his pain as though it were my own.

I did not realize until my adult years that my childhood ability to daydream would become a valuable asset in helping me navigate through some very difficult times. Perhaps I got some of my skill from my father. Although he had very little formal education, he was one of the smartest people I knew. He loved cutting out articles and pictures of places all over the world. He kept them in envelopes and folders where he could access them easily. He would study them carefully, satisfied that he had been there without ever venturing far from home. My father was contented with his life. He never desired more than he had and never struggled internally with the worry that he wasn't good enough. I admired and loved that part of him.

We had very little money for extras, but my dad always hid black licorice pieces in various locations around the house, giving us this very special treat when it was good and stale. I realized much later that he gave it to us when it was rock hard so that we could only eat a few pieces at a time and it would last much longer. My husband laughs at me because no matter where I travel in the world, I am always on the hunt for stale black licorice. There was something about my dad that drew me to him from a very early age. He used to ask the three of us if anyone wanted to go for a Sunday drive with him. The others always declined the invitation. I simply adored sitting beside him in the car. Often hours would pass without a word being exchanged. It didn't matter. Sometimes there is no need for words. Although he was not a big talker, he exuded love, and all I wanted to do was climb into his lap and settle there like a contented kitten. I felt safe and protected with him. Those were some of the qualities I would later look for in my husband.

I STILL REMEMBER the moment Jonathan and I met. It was my first day of university. I was very excited to be heading off to freshman orientation. I told my parents that I was going to become the world's greatest historian. My father laughed and told me that I was actually going to university to find a husband.

I walked barefoot into Sir George Williams University, now called Concordia University, wearing blue jeans and a silk shirt. I had long, straight dark hair. Of course, today I cringe when I think about walking downtown barefoot. I couldn't have cared less back then. I was a free spirit, and nothing bothered me.

I sat down beside my girlfriend Linda Carson. We were partners in crime and had been best friends since kindergarten. All of a sudden, Jonathan appeared in front of me. There was just something about him that made me weak in the knees. He wore a three-piece suit and was giving the welcoming address to all the freshmen. I was totally smitten. I turned to Linda and said, "See that guy over there? That is what I want!" He had a twinkle in his eye, and he exuded confidence. Little did I know that he also turned to his friend, pointed my way, and said, "See that Indian over there? I am going to ask her to have lunch with me!" To this day, I am still referred to jokingly as "Pocahontas."

Jonathan is a dreamer and a doer. I used to wonder if he ever slept. His mind is always tuned to building or fixing something. He faces challenges with great strength and gusto. There was a part of me that imagined him capable of handling any obstacle that crossed his path. It was always important for me to have a partner who could protect me and make me feel safe. Jon fit that bill.

After three years of dating on and off, Jonathan and I married. I guess my father was right after all. We had our wedding reception in the backyard of the home I had grown up in. Although it was small, I had always loved my house and dreamed of getting married there. I borrowed my cousin's wedding dress and had a beautiful afternoon ceremony with only the closest of friends and family. I spent the next two years finishing my university degree while Jon worked hard establishing himself in the business world. To the outside world, our family life appeared quite ordinary. To me, it was everything I had ever wanted.

From the time I was a little girl, I had dreamed of becoming a mother. I couldn't think of anything else I wanted to be. And from the moment I married Jon, at age twenty, I knew I was ready. Convincing him was another matter. I remember him telling me that starting a family was not like buying a dress. "If you don't like it, you can't just give it back," Jonathan used to quip. He told me that he had a five-year plan, to which I responded, "Stalin had a five-year plan too. His failed and yours is going to as well." The decision to have children was not made on a whim. It was something hardwired into my DNA.

Jonathan's plan did in fact fail, and Jacqueline was born two years later. The joy and privilege I felt at being able to stay home and raise her was beyond words. I recall spending the first three months of her life in awe of this little being. I ate, drank and slept her. There were many times when my husband had to remind me that we were a family of three, not two. Everything she did filled me with excitement. She was my entire world, and to me this felt like heaven.

My second daughter, Katherine, was born when I turned twenty-four years old. I had experienced a very difficult pregnancy. There had been an eighty-five percent chance that she would have severe mental deficits, and the doctors tried to discuss different institutional options with me. I felt myself sink into a dark hole, refusing to listen to them for fear of falling apart completely. I went into labor in my seventh month and remained in hospital on different medications and complete bed rest for more than two months. The guilt I felt for being away from Jacqueline was hard enough to bear, but the pain I experienced with the potential loss of Katherine was excruciating. It was a very difficult time for all three of us. Ultimately, she was born perfectly healthy, and I was on top of the world. I feared having any more children after that experience, but my doctor assured me that the complications that had occurred during my pregnancy with Kassy were very unlikely to be repeated.

I was grateful for my doctor's counsel, because until Alexandra was born, in February 1981, I never felt that my family was complete. She was the easiest baby, and I was beyond thrilled. Three beautiful little girls! I remember laughing out loud after I gave birth to Ali, telling Jon that I was sure the next one would be a boy. He looked me straight in the eye and said, "Four women for the rest of my life I can live with; five might push me right over the edge."

I was a very busy mom and, just like my mother, shouldered almost the entire responsibility for raising the girls. I never felt burdened by it and was so grateful for the opportunity to be able to stay home and take care of them. Jon worked endlessly, trying to build up a business from scratch so that he could support his family. From the time he was young, he had learned that there is no free ride in life. His parents made him understand very early that if he wanted anything, he would have to find a way to earn the money himself. He sacrificed much family time together to ensure that we were well looked after.

A few months before Kassy was born, Jon bought the house we would live in for the next thirty-seven years. I had grown up in a very small home and was shocked when I saw it. With tears in my eyes, I asked him how I could possibly clean such a large home and look after our family at the same time. He laughed and told me I could get someone to help me once in a while. This idea was foreign to me, and I was not sure I liked it. When I was growing up, we never had anyone come into our home to help us. If I had someone else clean my home, would that show that I couldn't handle my responsibilities on my own? What would my role be then? It seemed that I was going to have to make a lot more adjustments in my life than simply moving into a new home.

If I had any free time—when the girls were in school or Jon was babysitting them—I spent it ballet dancing and playing tennis. Ever since I was a child, I'd felt alive whenever I danced. When I was eight years old, I was recruited by Les Grands Ballets Canadiens. My mom sat me down and asked me how seriously I wanted to dance. I told her I wanted to simply enjoy it and not put in the kind of work that a career would require. When I got a little older, I trained with a Russian ballet company. I continued dancing until I was twenty-seven years old. When I danced, I could feel each and every muscle in my body working in unison. I felt as strong as Goliath and as free as a bird. Any problems I may have had were put on the back burner. When I was dancing, all there was room for in my brain was dance.

I learned to play tennis when I was at summer camp and took to it straight away. Jon and I still play regularly. I am not competitive by nature, but with a tennis racket in my hand and my husband across the court—watch out! I love the thrill of a great shot, and watching him struggle to return it is not too bad either. To this day, Jon is still afraid of me when I get close to the net. Somehow, he doesn't believe that I would never hit him on purpose.

IN MY LATE TWENTIES, I began to notice that I was having more aches and pains than I was used to. I had to stop dancing because my knees ached and filled with fluid whenever they were stressed. My back also hurt and felt tired much of the time. I decided that this was probably the result of carrying the kids around. I was pretty sure that fatigue must be a common complaint of most young mothers.

My late twenties and early thirties were challenging both physically and emotionally. Growing up, I had always been happy and content. I was innocent and very naive. I was that kid on the block everyone considered sweet. If one of my neighbors was baking cookies, I was welcomed into their home with open arms. I hated conflict and, even before the age of ten, claimed the role of mediator. My brother, not so kindly, labeled me "Sweet Sucky Susie." Sweet was never an act; I was a truly joyful person. One of the reasons I had children was to share with them the gladness I felt in simply being alive. I did not have any lofty goals other than living peacefully with my husband and my children.

Nevertheless, I found myself in a continuous conflict with my mother-in-law. Early in the marriage, things between us were great. I felt tremendous warmth and respect for her. She was very physical, and we enjoyed playing tennis, skiing, or biking together. From the time I had children, however, and did not raise them the way she would have liked me to, our relationship eroded. It was her way or the highway. One day, she came into my house and presented me with a written list of twenty-seven things she did not like about me. She thought she was being helpful, that it would somehow help me to be a better wife, mother, and of course daughter-in-law. I thought I would die. I couldn't even find the words to speak. I sat in my kitchen after she left and cried until my husband came home from work. I was totally crushed.

From that point, I was lost. My self-confidence and self-esteem seemed to crumble. I thought perhaps there was something wrong with me. I could not understand: Why did this woman turn against me? Her resentment was palpable. What did I ever do to deserve it? Couldn't she just be satisfied that my husband and children were happy and well looked after?

I became stuck. Years passed, but I could never move on. It didn't matter where I went or what I did, she was always in my head. In time, she took on the role of martyr (having delivered her version of the truth), and I chose that of victim. We both could have won Academy Awards for our performances. I blamed everyone for not helping me show her how wrong she was and how right I was. It is unbelievable how the fear (of not being liked or accepted) and guilt (maybe I really did something to merit this reaction), combined with a lack of self-confidence, held me back like a powerful magnet, binding me to a sick and destructive relationship. My mother had always taught me that it was better to say nothing if I had nothing nice to say about someone. But that was hard to do. I could never understand how this person, who supposedly loved me, could act so cruelly toward me. I held my tongue as I was taught, suffered in silence, and kept all my pain inside.

My physical aches and pains never did let up. In fact, they turned out to be more serious than I first thought. By the time I was thirty, I required knee reconstruction, and at thirty-two, spinal fusion of three discs because of my extensive ballet practice in my youth. If that wasn't enough, I also ended up requiring three abdominal laparoscopic surgeries, only to be followed by a hysterectomy, all before I was thirty-five.

I was one of the unlucky women who had a flawed "Copper-7" IUD placed inside them as a form of birth control. I developed pelvic inflammatory disease, which ultimately resulted in the removal of my uterus. Shortly after my ordeal, that type of IUD was taken off the market. Although it was hard on all of us having me in and out of hospital so often, I attributed all these events to bad luck and nothing more.

One of the things I had learned from being a dancer was discipline. I was good with my body. I was able to handle the surgeries like a real trooper, keeping my wits about me and doing whatever was necessary to ensure speedy recoveries. I rarely complained and was grateful that whatever was wrong with me was fixable. My family and friends (not including my mother-in-law) considered me a Wonder Woman.

Little did I know that my optimistic nature was about to be seriously challenged. When I awoke one fateful August morning, I was about to embark on a journey that would both change and reshape my life forever.

(2)

UPON DIAGNOSIS

IT WAS MID-AUGUST 1989. I was just thirty-six years old. Jacqueline was almost fourteen, Kassy was twelve, and Alexandra was eight. Jonathan and I had been married for more than fifteen years. The characteristics that had attracted me to him more than eighteen years earlier were still evident each and every day of our lives.

Jon and I were holidaying with friends in Vancouver, while the girls were still away at summer camp. All of us would be returning home within a few days. A trip to the bathroom left me shaken. As soon as I saw blood on the toilet paper, a sickening knowing flooded me. I tried to pull myself together. I remembered having had a similar experience with hemorrhoids a few months prior. They were tied off, and my doctor told me not to worry. She explained that they were sometimes a result of childbirth. I accepted her explanation with little hesitation. But this time something was different. I just couldn't seem to convince myself that I was okay. In that moment, looking at the toilet paper covered in blood, my body knew. Every cell screamed "cancer!" I tried desperately to separate my head from my body. "Let's not jump the gun," I told myself.

Eight years earlier, when I was twenty-eight, I had taken a training course with a palliative care team headed by Dr. Balfour Mount at the Royal Victoria Hospital in Montreal. We underwent six months of classroom instruction and three months of training on the floor to see whether we would be able to handle dealing with patients who were dying. I loved learning from so many wonderful people, such as Elisabeth Kübler-Ross, who were experts in their field. We were trained to help the nurses in all aspects of patient care, and the nurses and doctors alike respected our contribution.

A nurse took me aside one day and told me that we were going to enter the room of a very sick woman. She warned me that the patient literally smelled as though she was rotting, and many found it difficult to work with her. I could tell by the odor as we walked down the hallway that we were close by. I walked over to the patient, introduced myself, and embraced her. As soon as I touched her, she started to cry in my arms. I wondered how long it must have been since anyone had held this woman. It was only after I left her room that I realized I had smelled nothing as soon as her eyes met mine.

Each patient I spoke to during my time working in palliative care told me that somewhere, deep inside, they knew that they were sick long before their doctors confirmed it. "Oh my God," I thought now, eight years later. "Is it possible I am now one of those people?" I was reminded of a young man I used to visit in the hospital as a volunteer. I asked him whether there was anything I could do to make him feel better. He then asked me whether I could cure his cancer. After I said no, he told me to get the hell out of his room. I left with my tail between my legs and wondered if I would ever truly be able to understand a cancer patient without having experienced the disease myself.

Was it possible that I unconsciously brought this upon myself? Did I actually *need* this experience to continue to work in this field? These thoughts made me feel worse. Back when I had first started working in palliative care, Jon asked if it was possible to catch cancer from the patients. He did not want me to embark on a career that could potentially threaten my life or the lives of the kids. I thought his worries were ridiculous then, but now I was not so sure.

"Jon, where are you?" I cried as I went to find him. I told him about the blood and what I feared it meant. "Please, please, can't you fix this, like you fix everything else?" With tears in his eyes, he just looked at me, saying nothing as he wrapped his arms around me. Jon tried his best to comfort me, but I was inconsolable. The facts of my young age, healthy lifestyle, and lack of family history of cancer did not make me feel better.

When I called the doctor from Vancouver and described my symptoms, I was scheduled for a colonoscopy a few days after my return home. A colonoscopy is a test that scopes the entire colon. A tube is inserted rectally, after an extensive colon cleanse. A camera inside the tube examines the tissue, and the doctor is then able to perform a biopsy, if need be.

A gnawing fear started building inside me. My carefree holiday had come to an abrupt end in the blink of an eye. I couldn't wait to get home. On one hand, the next few days seemed to move at a snail's pace; on the other hand, they went far too quickly.

FINALLY, WE WERE all home. The girls were happily chatting together, filling us in on all the camp stories. I found myself half-listening at best. I found it amazing how I could be in two places at the same time. Physically, I was there, pretending to be involved and interested in what they were telling me. Mentally and emotionally, though, I was far away. "This can't be happening to me," I thought. I felt a black cloud surround me, and I found functioning normally next to impossible.

I asked my father to take me to the hospital for the colonoscopy a few days later. Jon was called out of town for an emergency business deal, which I thought was a sign of good karma. When you are scared and desperate, everything is a possible sign! I was so nervous. I could almost hear my heart, it was beating so furiously. Could I be overreacting? Was it possible that I was just a drama queen and this was really nothing, or could my days be numbered?

I was grateful that the waiting would soon be over. I needed to get to the bottom of this. When I arrived at the hospital, I kissed my father on both cheeks, gave him a hug, and said that I would see him soon. I was hooked up to an IV and given a combination of Valium and Demerol both to ease the pain from the procedure and to relax me. Wow! When the drugs kicked in, I felt as though I was floating. What an incredible feeling. I remember thinking that this must be the reason people do drugs. That magical feeling, however, was short-lived.

My doctor was a woman named Carol-Ann Vasilevsky. I had met her only once before, but as soon as she called for a biopsy tray, I knew my life was in her hands. She had seen a polyp growing through the muscle into the wall of the colon. The bleeding that had brought me to the hospital was purely coincidental. It had come from internal hemorrhoids. "Thank goodness," the doctor said. But whether the polyp was cancerous or not, I would be having surgery. She explained to me that a polyp growing into the lining of the colon was potentially more serious than one growing into the actual colon passage.

The deeper it infiltrates, the greater chance it has of pene-
trating the colon wall. And if that happens, the likelihood of
cancer spreading increases exponentially.

The date was August 23, 1989. Jon's birthday was on the
25th. The 26th was our anniversary. Carol-Ann had just
received a cancellation, and so she scheduled me for admis-
sion to the hospital on the 27th. Once again, I felt that things
were moving far too quickly. "Wait!" I screamed. "We don't
even know if it is cancer." Carol-Ann promised to have the
results of the biopsy in the next few days but insisted the
surgery was not optional. "There is no time to wait," she said
with certainty.

Time stopped. Breath stopped. Emotion stopped. I couldn't
speak. I couldn't think. Carol-Ann told me to rest for an hour,
and then she would come back to talk to me before I went
home. Forget that. I needed to get the hell out of there. There
was no way I was going to wait even another minute. All of
a sudden I felt trapped, like a caged animal. I had to leave as
quickly as possible. The effects of the drugs vanished in a second. I dressed mechanically and went out into the waiting
room to find my dad.

His initial smile turned into a look of alarm when he
saw my face. My words must have ripped out his heart. "She
thinks I may have cancer, Daddy," was all I could say. My father
wrapped his arms around me as he led me to the car. Neither
of us spoke the entire ride home. I could not remember ever
feeling this way before. I was completely emotionally flat. I
couldn't speak, because there was absolutely nothing to say.
My dad was also silent. He must have known that if he spoke,
the wave of emotion he unleashed would be so powerful that it
might drown us both.

Human beings are a funny species. We often react in strange ways to stressful circumstances. You might imagine I would have wanted to be surrounded by my closest friends and family members, to be comforted and nurtured by them. Nope, not me. In fact, I wanted nothing to do with anyone. "Leave me alone," was all I could think. The idea of anyone feeling sorry for me might have unglued me in an instant. I needed to do everything I could simply to function. I needed to protect myself. I distanced myself from everyone and everything. I refused to answer the telephone, knowing that if my mom called I might start to cry and never stop. I waited until the girls got home from visiting their friends, put food in a cooler, got into the car, and went with my daughters to hide out in the safety of my country cottage. There was a small part of me that was still hoping cancer couldn't find me there. I had never, after all, given it my address.

THE NEXT FEW days were excruciating. I refused to let Jon come home from Toronto. I assured him, in my usual manner, that I was fine. If it was cancer, I would need him later, not now. For the moment, I was untouchable. I did not want to be hugged or coddled. I just needed my space. I thought I had done an expert job at appearing to keep it together. Little did I know that my demeanor gave off a completely different message.

The girls told me afterwards that my behavior had made them extremely fearful. They knew something was up and did their best to keep out of my hair, as much for their own protection as for mine. I sat outside on our back balcony, staring at the lake, with the telephone resting on my lap. I was paralyzed with fear as I waited for it to ring. It never did.

On the afternoon of the second day, as I sat with the phone on the balcony and the children played across the street, suddenly, my husband appeared. He approached me tenderly, but his body language gave my diagnosis away. I knew I was in trouble as soon as I saw his slumped shoulders and the deep sadness in his eyes. But all I could focus on was my anger. What was wrong with my doctor? How dare she call Jon before me? That must be what she'd done—why else would he have flown home from Toronto and driven an hour out of the city without calling me? Didn't I have the right to hear the news first? I am not a baby. It was *my* cancer after all. There I was, sitting like an idiot, glued to the phone, afraid to even go to the bathroom for fear of missing the call. Logically, I knew that she did not want me to be alone when I found out. At that moment, however, logic was unimportant. No explanation was good enough. Only when my husband said that he needed to be the one to tell me, not some doctor, did I finally understand.

He asked me not to tell the girls until we both had time to digest the news and figure out an action plan. I realize he was trying to protect them, but not telling them made no sense to me. I refused to listen to him. The girls were not stupid. Why would Daddy appear in the country in the middle of the week if something was not seriously wrong? It was not like he did this on a regular basis. Nondisclosure would be like lying. They needed to know. I was shocked when he fell to the ground, crying and pounding the earth. I stood there with my mouth open, wondering why he was being so dramatic when I was the one with cancer. He must have felt impotent in his inability to shield and protect all of us from the pain that lay ahead. I felt sorry for him but knew that it didn't matter what he thought. I was going to do what I knew to be right. At that moment, the control Jon may have felt he was losing was my gain.

———

I HAVE ALWAYS found solace in writing. It allows me to go quietly into my heart and express emotion that is sometimes too difficult for me to share with anyone else.

Despair
Oh, wailing heart
Where do you go in the darkest of nights?
When even the wind turns it back on you?
The sun's warmth feels like hot cinders upon your skin;
The coolness of the moon chills the life force from your lungs.
All you have ever imagined, gone with just a few words.
And yet the power of those words is like a dagger to your soul.
Real and yet so surreal.
Yesterday all was normal,
Cooking, shopping, and tending to chores.
Filling some of the mundaneness of life.
Time, often endless, has new meaning.
Hope changes from fanciful imagining to desperate prayer.
All that was known is gone.
All that was innocent evaporates.
A moment in time
Changes all of a lifetime.

———

My poor husband tried to reassure me. What good would that do, I wondered? Nothing he did could change the pathology results. He tried to hold me, but I was already gone. I couldn't feel anything. I was getting used to this strange sense of numbness. It was weird but interesting. I could just go through the motions. I simply couldn't feel anything.

Jon told me that we needed to get the kids and pack up the house. Carol-Ann wanted me in the hospital for testing early the next morning. He went to get the girls, and when they returned, the aura of doom and gloom that surrounded the four of them took my breath away. They could barely look me in the eye. I stood there and bluntly told my daughters that I had cancer. I felt their hugs embrace my body and their tears seep deeply into my soul. Jon joined in the group hug, holding our daughters close as they cried, united in shock and fear. I could not cry. I just stood there. Eventually, I peeled them off my body, packed up the few things I had brought with me, and drove home. I have no idea whether I drove home alone or with the kids. That moment is gone from my memory banks forever.

There are some things that are too painful to be remembered. I think that the automatic pilot part of us takes over. In retrospect, I believe that an innate protective mechanism exists within all of us. It is that part that seems to know exactly how much we can handle. Anything more could push us over the edge. Numbness and memory blanks were becoming a protective strategy. Too many things were happening at once for me to deal with. Blissful disappearance became a coping tool.

(3)

INTO THE ABYSS

IT JUST SO happened that my oldest and dearest friend, Linda, was in town because her mother had recently been diagnosed with breast cancer. Talk about timing! The next morning, I found myself in the hospital with Jon, Linda, and her husband, Stephen, by my side. Stephen is a pediatric pulmonologist, and it felt good having him there not only for moral support but also to explain things to me if I could not understand them. X-rays, scans, and blood tests seemed to be the order of the day. I felt like a lab rat being poked and prodded.

Once the tests were complete, Carol-Ann told me with great relief that the preliminary testing appeared to show that the cancer was contained. I was glad she was relieved; I, on the other hand, sat there, completely stunned. What had she just said? I am an intelligent person and a university graduate. Why then had the possibility of a metastatic disease never even occurred to me? What was she not telling me? What else had she seen when she scoped me? Had she suspected more cancer? Could death really be knocking on my door? Her words felt like knives stabbing at my heart. I was overwhelmed by the idea that she was even looking to see if the cancer had spread elsewhere. I sat there, frozen like a statue, paralyzed and in shock.

Somehow, Jon, Linda, and Stephen managed to take over and get me home. If someone had asked me to describe myself at that moment, I would have said "an empty shell." I felt lost in an abyss of nothingness. I was a mere robot that walked and talked, devoid of anything that made me feel human. What a horrible day it had been. Happy birthday to you, Jon. My present for you this year is my living nightmare.

The next day was our sixteenth wedding anniversary. When I awoke that morning, I wondered if I would ever have another. Jon tried to do something nice. He prepared a picnic basket and off we went to the port in Old Montreal. He then did the unforgivable. I became hysterical as soon as he took the movie camera out of the car. "This is not *Love Story*!" I shrieked. "Do you think I'm going to die, so you need to film today as a keepsake?" I really upset him and the girls. No matter what he did, it was wrong. My poor little girls cowered around their father for support. They were too terrified to come close to me, and who could blame them?

My sister and her family took us out for dinner that evening to celebrate our anniversary. Growing up, Linda had always been the sibling Stephen and I would go to in times of trouble. She was more of a mother to us than a big sister. Her job seemed to be to take care of us. Here she was, doing whatever she could to normalize a situation that was anything but normal. Everyone appeared to be having a good time, but I became aware that something very strange was happening. Everyone was talking and laughing, but all I could hear were muffled sounds. It felt as though someone had put their hands tightly over my ears. No matter how hard I tried, I could not hear words clearly. What was happening to me now? Why weren't my ears working? Did they decide on their own that they could not bear to hear any more bad news, so they just shut down? Were they trying to protect me? I wondered if I had already begun unconsciously to separate from those around me.

I was reminded of a nature program I had seen on television in which the sick animal left its family to wander away alone to die. Is this what was happening? So far, I thought I had done a somewhat reasonable job of keeping sane. Now I was no longer sure. This felt completely out of my control. Then my food came. I had no recollection of even ordering anything. I tasted it, and it was horrible. "Oh my God," I thought. "Now my taste buds aren't working either!" I burst into tears, ran to the bathroom, and threw up. This was all too much for me to take. Dinner was over. It was time to go home.

There were only three nights between diagnosis and surgery. It seemed to be just enough time for each of my daughters to have a nightmare. Ali did not remember the specifics of her dream, only that she felt scared. My heart ached for my little peanut. By the time she was two years old, I had begun having one surgery after another. She spent so much time upstairs in my bedroom, coloring or doing her homework in bed beside me. All she had ever known since her birth was that Mommy was upstairs, recovering from one of her many operations. How unfair this was for her. When my spine was fused, I was forced to wear a body brace for six months. In order to get a simple hug from me, she needed to climb up onto my lap. I wasn't even able to bend down and pick up my little girl.

Jacqueline's nightmare came next. She told me with tears pouring down her face that she had dreamed I died in a car crash, not from cancer. We talked for more than an hour. Afterwards, she hugged me and said that she had decided she would handle everything at home and I should not worry about the girls. Was she taking over my role? Imagine that: my almost-fourteen-year-old would be "fixing" everything at home instead of wondering who her next boyfriend would be.

Around 2 a.m. that same night, it was Kassy's turn. She dreamed that she was the one who had cancer, lost all her hair, and was going to die. We talked until about three, when she finally asked, "What would I ever do without you, Mom? If you die, who will make me feel as good about myself as you have?" I reassured her that I would be around for a very long time... but would I?

Her question broke my heart. On one hand, the girls gave me the gift of reminding me how much I was loved and why I needed to get well. On the other, I felt that a huge burden of responsibility was on my shoulders to ensure not only my well-being but theirs as well. None of us knows for sure what future challenges might befall us. God only knows how unprepared I was for what I was about to face. How was I going to get through this? Would there be enough time for me to prepare them for the possibility of life without me? Could I take care of them properly while trying to take care of myself? I still had so much work to do, and my girls needed me. I told them that although I could not promise them I would never get sick again, I could promise that I was not done living yet. My goal became to make my daughters as strong and independent as I possibly could.

Eventually, the girls all fell asleep in their beds. No one was having an easy time knowing that I would be entering the hospital the next morning. I turned to Jon, looked deeply into his eyes, and we made desperate love. I think I was trying to make sure that there was a part of me that was still alive and could feel something. I drank in every ounce of his being, hoping that he would somehow supplement my depleting energy resources.

Before I left my house the next day, I looked in the mirror and wondered if I would ever be coming home. Would I be the same Susan who left? I already couldn't recognize myself. Those weren't my eyes looking back at me in the mirror. I had become a stranger to myself. How had that happened so quickly? All I did was function. I was just a body, existing. I wasn't even scared at that moment. Feeling scared required energy, and I had very little left.

THE SURGICAL PREPARATIONS were arduous, as the colon is quite the dirty organ. It must be meticulously cleaned and emptied before surgery, so as to avoid infection. Psychologically, I was not ready for all the preparation. I had gone through it just a few days earlier for the colonoscopy, and look what the result had been. Just the idea of taking the cleanse traumatized me. The nurses were annoyed with me. I was not being a very compliant patient. They told me that I had no choice but to take the colon cleanse. Just the thought of drinking that stuff made me sick to my stomach. The mind can be very powerful, and mine was definitely getting in the way. Thank goodness my friend Linda's husband, Stephen, came to the rescue. He was able to hypnotize me so that I could drink the gallon of saline solution. A part of me will always associate it with the diagnosis of cancer.

Jon, Linda, and Stephen hovered, trying to be helpful, but I couldn't stand it. I asked them all to leave. The idea of having anyone there trying to comfort me was irritating. Was this a show? Was my personal horror meant to be shared? My soul was crying, and my spirit was cracking. This was not the life I signed up for, and I certainly did not want the leading role in this drama. I became very small and childlike. Where was the strong woman, the protective wife and mother who would fight to the death for her family? In that moment, I realized she was gone. I began to wonder if she would ever come back. Could I ever learn to fight for myself?

Jon arranged to have a nurse spend the night before the surgery and a few nights afterwards with me. He needed to be at home with the girls and didn't want me to be alone. To remain sane, he needed to know that I was well looked after. This was perfectly fine with me, since I so desperately needed my privacy and space. I couldn't stand the thought of anyone walking on eggshells around me, feeling horrible for my situation. I had enough to deal with. I arranged with the nurses that when I pretended to fall asleep, it was time to ask visitors to leave. This was a perfect arrangement. No one's feelings would be hurt, and my needs would be met.

Eventually, after eighteen hours, all the preparations were over. I was exhausted, depleted, and done. It was well after midnight, and I wondered if sleep would be possible. I must have dozed, because all of a sudden, Jon and the girls were there wishing me well. I hugged them until it hurt. I told them how much I loved them and then asked everyone to leave. The ache of having them there, reminding me of what I might lose, was too painful for me at that moment.

Finally, the floodgates opened. Fear flowed out of every pore in my body. I could not keep it together any longer. I wept for what felt like an eternity. Then an orderly came to get me. What a lonely and weird little trip it was to the operating room. I remember thinking that the walls of the hospital corridor needed to be painted. It all seemed surreal and dreamlike. The operating room was freezing cold. I felt like a slab of meat about to be butchered. Everyone was busy hurrying about, readying themselves for the big event.

Suddenly, I started to shiver uncontrollably. I was terrified. I started to cry. I then felt a hand on my shoulder. I looked up and our eyes locked. Carol-Ann gazed at me with such kindness that I immediately felt safe. She was only thirty-three years old, and I was thirty-six. Before falling asleep, I remember thinking that maybe we would grow old together.

UPON AWAKENING, I felt pain. I thought that this was good. I was very familiar with pain. "I am alive," I thought. "I'll get through this."

Carol-Ann was very pleased with the results from the surgery. She had removed six inches of colon on either side of the polyp and then stitched the colon back together again. She removed the ovary that was nearby, fearing the possibility of its having cancer as well. It is pretty amazing to think that doctors can simply cut out pieces of your body and put them back together again. No matter how many different operations I've been through, I am in awe of the body's capacity to heal itself. It doesn't seem to matter how many things we remove or alter. We are able to keep on going. The human body is truly remarkable!

Although the surgery had gone well and statistics suggested I had a ninety-five percent chance of disease-free living, a consultation with an oncologist was set up. The pathologist had found that the polyp was a Dukes B2. Dukes is a staging system for colon cancer. Dukes A is generally when the cancer stays in the innermost lining of the colon or rectum. Dukes B is when the cancer has grown through the muscle layer. Mine had gone right to the edge, hence the number 2. Dukes C means that the cancer has spread to at least one lymph node. I think we all can figure out what Dukes D, or stage four, means.

The results of the pathology were sent to a tumor board for review. The tumor board consists of doctors in radiotherapy, surgery, internal medicine, and pathology, as well as psychosocial specialists. After reviewing my case, the group decided on what they felt would be the best course of treatment for me. Because of my age and the fact that the cancer had gone into the muscle wall, they recommended chemotherapy. Had they told me to jump off a bridge with the promise that it would make me better, I would have agreed. I was very vulnerable. I didn't want to die. "Give me a pill, a promise, a guarantee, I'm in!" I thought.

Although I never questioned my treatment plan, my mother certainly did. She wanted to know why I would "put poison" into my body if I didn't really need it; after all, a ninety-five-percent chance of disease-free living without it was pretty good odds. I did not have an answer to give her at the time. But as I pondered this question, I thought that if cancer ever came back, even five years later, and I had not done chemotherapy, would I be able to live with myself? Would I blame myself for missing an opportunity that might have potentially been helpful? I did not ever want to be in that position. In hindsight, I think having chemotherapy was easier than wishing I had done it. I had worked with cancer patients as a volunteer for eight years before my diagnosis. Most of them had experienced some form of chemotherapy, and many had survived it. I hoped it wouldn't be too difficult to endure.

I was told that one side effect of the treatment would be thinning hair (not great, since I had baby-fine hair to start with), but I was reassured that I would not lose it all. I was upset when a nurse from the oncology department suggested that I buy a wig, just in case I lost more hair than was expected.

When Jon saw how upset I was about that possibility, he told me I was being "overly dramatic and superficial." I hated him for saying that. Superficial is something I have never and will never be. The idea of losing my hair versus losing my life was a no-brainer for either of us, but for me, my hair had a very different meaning. My hair was a form of protection. It saved me from being exposed to the world. Did everyone really need to know that I was dealing with cancer? My hair gave me a sense of anonymity. This was much more than mere vanity. I had lost so much of my footing already. When I looked in the mirror and saw my thinning hair, I was reminded of how I could not escape my circumstances. To Jon, it was no big deal. But I wonder how he would really have felt if I had walked around bald at one of his business functions. Once again, unless it is happening to you, it is very hard to really understand. In the end, I lost about a third of my hair, and I never wore the wig.

I had a mini-breakdown three days after surgery, alone in my room in the dead of night. "It's not fair," I told myself. "I eat so well, I exercise, I'm optimistic. Was there more I could have done to stop this from happening? How can I have what is often referred to as the 'ultimate failure of the body's immune system'?" I did not like this expression from the first time I heard it, when I was working in palliative care. What did I do to make my immune system fail? Was this really possible? I was so young. I thought I had taken such good care of myself.

What a joke! I must have been completely delusional. I know now that taking care of myself is not just about eating well or exercising regularly. Psychological, emotional, and spiritual well-being have to combine with physical well-being for ultimate health. I will never know if I might have changed the course of my life had I been more aware of the fact that I was harming myself by keeping pain, sadness, and frustration alive deep down in my gut. I would like to think, however, that by being more aware now, I have a better chance of dealing with difficult or uncomfortable issues before they can potentially harm me.

Wouldn't you know it, but just as the floodgates opened for a second time, Carol-Ann walked into the room. She had come to the hospital after an evening event, all dressed up, simply to check on her patients. She sat down on the edge of my bed and asked the nurse to leave so that we could talk privately. Although she was so young, she seemed to have the wisdom of someone far beyond her years. Perhaps that's what working in oncology does; it makes you see more clearly. It was hard for me to put my thoughts into words. After I mumbled my complaints about how unfair life was, she stood up, ripped the blankets from my bed, and lifted up my dressing gown. "Have a good look at the scar on your belly," she said. "It usually takes three weeks for the stitches to heal as well as they have in three days." She reminded me that a healthy body recovers much better and faster than an unhealthy one. "Stop feeling sorry for yourself," she reprimanded. "Your prognosis is excellent. Now get on with living!" Although I hated the look of my belly post-surgery, I hoped that my vanity would not get the better of me. Never wearing a bikini again would not be so terrible. No one, other than Jon and me, ever had to see what really lay beneath my clothing. A few lumps and bumps were a small price to pay for having beaten cancer.

I had a ninety-five percent chance of disease-free living. It was time to get into action and create some sort of a plan for living. Carol-Ann had given me the kick I needed. It was amazing to have a doctor willing to go that extra mile. Her care went above and beyond anything I might have expected, and I appreciated it so much. It was Carol-Ann's eyes that had comforted me just before surgery, and here she was again, saving me, but this time from myself. I truly did have an angel by my side. For whatever reason, fate had put us together, and nothing was going to pull us apart. She was my anchor from the start, and I am grateful that she is still a part of my life to this day.

The next morning, I met with my oncologist, Alex Zukiwski, for the first time. He had just arrived in Montreal from MD Anderson Cancer Center in Houston, Texas. He was young and seemed kind and genuinely concerned. I developed an instant rapport with him. During one of our appointments, another doctor knocked on the door and opened it up to ask him a question. After a few more interruptions, Alex got up, locked the door, and refused to speak to anyone other than me. "This is not a cold," he said emphatically. "You deserve all the time you need to have your questions answered without interruption." How sad that this attitude is not commonplace.

He told me that chemotherapy would begin three weeks after surgery. He wanted to eliminate the chance of even one hidden cancer cell coming back to get me in the future. It sounded good to me. I realized after he left my hospital room that I did not even ask a single question. I normally had a lot to say about a lot of things. Why was I speechless then? It did not matter that I had worked with oncology patients as a volunteer since I was twenty-eight years old. I was still totally unprepared when cancer happened to me. Today, I would have an entire book filled with questions at a meeting like that. Back then, I thought anything anyone said was all right. All I wanted was for someone to take over and make me better. At that moment, I had no idea what I could possibly do to help myself. It had all happened too quickly. There had been less than a week between diagnosis and surgery. I had no time to prepare. I therefore put all of my trust in my medical team.

TIME PASSED AND I began to heal. Finally, about ten days after surgery, I was ready to go home. I couldn't wait to jump back into my old life. I was more excited than a child at an amusement park. Jon came to get me, and we chatted happily all the way home. I could not wait to see my kids.

My dog greeted me like a long-lost lover when I walked in the door, not leaving my side even for a second. This little being had been so depressed by my disappearance that my family had to sneak her into the hospital to see me just to get her to start eating again. It felt so nice to receive this kind of unconditional love. It's funny; I am not really a dog person. I care about animals in general, but until I rescued this little dog, Scruffy, I never understood what it meant to really love a pet. No matter what mood I was in, or how upset I may have been, just being near her was tonic for my soul.

Everything else at home was weird. I returned expecting to find chaos. After all, the central household figure had just been in hospital for more than a week, with a diagnosis of cancer, no less! To my astonishment, all seemed to be perfectly in order. The girls were at school, the house was spotless, the fridge was full, and the laundry had been done. All household duties had been delegated, and Jon managed with the rest. The least functional member of my family was my dog. "Thank goodness for her," I thought. At least someone appeared to be suffering from my absence. In a way, this was a rude awakening. It was the first time in my life that I realized I was dispensable. The world did not fall apart because I was gone.

This was an incredibly pivotal moment in my life. It was not frightening as much as it was awakening for me. Did I really think that everyone else's life would stop because mine had? Was my sense of self so falsely inflated? I felt like a balloon that had just had all the air taken out of it. My whole life revolved around taking care of my family. It was my job and a role that I had always loved and wanted. What if I didn't make it? What if I was in that fifth percentile? I saw that my family managed just fine. Perhaps they were sad, perhaps even scared, but the reality was that life was going on for them just the same. Everything I had counted on, everything I thought I knew for certain, was gone. I felt as though I was purposeless. I could not understand how everything in my family's lives had gone on as though nothing was different, while everything in my life had changed in the blink of an eye. Nothing would ever be the same for me again. I wondered how a paradigm shift of such magnitude could happen so quickly, yet I felt as though I was the only one affected by it.

I found myself irritable. My normally relaxed disposition was anything but. Everything bothered me, and I had no patience for small talk. I remember how my aunt avoided me because of her discomfort in dealing with a "cancer patient." Finally, she got up the nerve to ask me how she should talk to me. "The same way you talked to me before," I barked back at her. I was still Susan, somewhere inside this shell of a person. People tried to be nice, but I didn't feel nice. They told me not to worry, that my prognosis was great. I wanted to scream. How stupid could they be? How dare they assume they could foresee my future? Just because the tumor was cut out, did that mean it was really gone? How did it get there in the first place? Why didn't I have any awareness of such an invader? What was wrong with me? Cancer doesn't just happen in a minute. It needs time to nurture itself, to grow, and to invade. How dare they tell me not to worry? It was not their body this was happening to.

Cancer is a strange disease. You would think that it might pull people closer together. Everyone participates in the helpful dance. They make meals, they run errands, and they take care of stuff. Now, don't get me wrong. All of that is important. It allows the household to function and maintains some sense of normalcy. What family and friends cannot do, however, is fill the empty space around the cancer patient. It was as though I was surrounded by a moat, and only those who had actually experienced the disease firsthand could come anywhere close. Everyone else remained across the water. I finally understood why the man I visited in palliative care had thrown me out of his room. I was absolutely not the kind of help he needed then. This disease separates people. I felt different from others, and when I was in the "poor me" stage, I resented the fact that not only were they healthy, but their lives were continuing as they always had. I felt very much alone and lost in the realization that nothing would ever be the same for me again. I experienced a loss of self and a sense of isolation with my diagnosis. "How can I get through this?" I asked myself. "Will I ever be able to make sense of how or why this happened to me? Will I ever feel safe in my skin again? How do I even begin to heal?"

(4)

FINDING FAITH

I HAD NEVER been a particularly religious person. Growing up, we were never encouraged to go to synagogue. It was deemed more important to learn the origins and traditions of Judaism than the spiritual principles of the faith: we celebrated the holidays that brought friends and family together. It was difficult to discuss the concept of "God" with my father. His beliefs were unyielding. "There could never be a 'God' who would allow such horrible things to have happened to so many people," he would say of the Holocaust. Although my father's family was untouched by the war, a large portion of my mother's family in Poland was killed by the Nazis. My father gained no comfort from religion and held his beliefs firmly until the day he died. My mother, however, did believe in God. But her principles were not necessarily rooted in any specific religion. Her values were more humanistic in nature. She believed in welcoming everyone into her home with respect and kindness.

After marrying Jon and having children, I never felt a strong desire to go to synagogue. But we went, because I felt that we owed it to our children to teach them about our culture. That way, they would at least have some sort of foundation to build upon should they desire to embrace our religion when they became adults.

Within a few days of leaving the hospital, it was time to celebrate the Jewish High Holidays. These holidays are regarded as the most important ones in Judaism. When I told Jon I had decided to go to synagogue, he asked me if I was sure. I had just been diagnosed with cancer. I would have to face so many people, and he did not want any of them saying anything that might upset me. I really appreciated his concern and knew that this was his way of trying to shield me from gawking eyes and wagging tongues. But I didn't care. Something was driving me there. It was not just a want; it was a need.

This time, I was being pulled toward the synagogue for a different reason. Something inside me thirsted for answers and desperately wanted some sort of peace. As we drove there, I asked the girls to sit quietly beside one another. My heart was pounding and sweat poured down my armpits, from both fear and general weakness. I anticipated that something important was going to happen there. When we entered the sanctuary, I held on to Jon's arm, and with the girls close by, I lowered my eyes and found my seat. Ultimately, it didn't matter how many people were there. I did not notice even a single one.

During the service, the rabbi discussed aspects of forgiveness, which is the central theme of the holiday Yom Kippur. We ask to be forgiven for any injury or wrongdoing we may have caused another. We also ask to find the ability to forgive those who may have harmed us in any way. Then and there, I decided that this was something I needed to do. I needed to forgive my mother-in-law, who had caused me so much harm, because her actions had been eating me alive. She had closed the door on me. Either I would behave in the manner she found acceptable, or we were not going to have a relationship. I had never been in a situation like this before, where someone didn't like me because I did not do what they wanted. I internalized all my frustration and often questioned myself. Perhaps I felt that on some level it was my inability to deal with her that may have contributed to my getting sick in the first place. Author Louise Hay suggests that, metaphysically, cancer is believed to result from a deep hurt, a deep grief eating away at you. The colon represents our ability to let go and release that which is no longer needed. I was definitely having trouble letting go.

Because I had absolutely no power to change my mother-in-law (let alone even discuss my feelings with her), I decided on a different approach. I needed to change the way I thought about her. I decided to start by giving the word "forgiveness" a new definition. I would not forget the past, for the past has always provided information that helps create the present. It was not about excusing or pardoning bad behaviors, because we need to remember not to do those things that may be hurtful to others. I decided that forgiveness for me would be about letting go. I could choose to let go of all those things that were causing me pain, and the trauma she'd caused was definitely one of those things! I needed to take back my power and start protecting myself. Jon couldn't fix this for me. I was the one who needed to learn to find my voice and fight for myself. I was determined to do this, because I desperately needed to focus all my strength on healing. I found my precious energy was leaking like water from a watering can. I needed to plug up all those holes through which it was seeping out. I could no longer occupy my mind, body, or soul with anything else. It was time to let go of the old stuff, change the story, and move forward.

The rabbi then read that it is God who decides who shall be sick or who shall be well, who shall live or who shall die. I remember hearing an internal scream so loud emanating from my gut: "Not my God!" I refused to believe that it was solely up to God to decide my fate. Didn't I have any role in determining the outcome of my destiny? If God was going to become an integral part of my healing process, then there would have to be a partnership between us. I was not going to give myself totally up to him; we would need to work together. I figured that it was up to me to decide what I was looking for. My challenge was to create a concept of God that would suit my needs.

I closed my eyes and remembered that when I was a girl, I loved placing my tiny little hand in my father's great big paw. The moment I did it, I felt safe and protected and whole. As I thought about this, I could feel a smile crease my face. When I looked up into my dad's eyes, they twinkled back at me like bright stars on a dark night. There was no judgment in those eyes. They shone with pure love and reflected back to me a sea of endless potential. I remember feeling in those moments that I was perfect exactly as I was and that I could do or be anything I set my mind to. This was exactly what I was looking for.

I had thought that constructing a personal concept of God was going to be an arduous process, but this was going better than I had anticipated. I began laying a foundation. I first needed the feeling of safety and protection. I had felt so lost and ungrounded following the diagnosis of cancer that I wanted to imagine my heart and soul held and rocked tenderly in the arms of God. I also needed to embrace the idea of limitless potential and no judgment.

I remember years later, when I had a counseling practice of my own, talking to a client of mine who was dying. She felt that she was damned and going to hell because she had converted to a religion she always felt should have been hers from birth. Now that she was dying, she was terrified that her choices would undermine her and that she would be sent to hell. She told me that she wanted my God, a God that was kind and forgiving. How sad that during her last moments on earth, religion was a source of terror for her. I had always thought that people turned to religion in the hope of being comforted. I determined it would be that way for me. Since I was making it up, I could do whatever I wanted. Little did I know that when I left the synagogue that day, God was going to become my constant companion and best friend for life.

———

· *finding solace* ·

ALTHOUGH I CAME from a background where religion did not play a profound role, I managed to find tremendous support and comfort in the concept of God. *Merriam-Webster's Collegiate Dictionary* defines faith as a "firm belief in something for which there is no proof." I have found that the word "faith" often substitutes for "hope." People who are not particularly spiritual or religious seem to pray for help when they feel threatened or when their loved ones are in dire straits. It is almost like wishing upon a star, hoping that somehow, someone out there might hear them and come to their rescue.

I needed to believe in something when I was sick. Because I had no idea whether I would live or die, I was looking for support irrespective of outcome. For that reason, I chose that which is intangible. It was important for me to find something that could not be touched or grasped. I needed to be able to wonder and dive into a world of possibility where no one could tell me for sure that what I chose to believe in was not real.

I found comfort in the notion of God. I did not expect him to alter the course of my life or take away my hurts and pain. What I wanted was to know that I did not have to walk this journey all by myself. I decided to personify God because it was easier for me to imagine communicating with him this way. I chose the idea of being held and rocked in the arms of God the same way my dad held me, and the way I in turn held and rocked my children when they were young. I remembered the pure joy and contentment I felt when I held them. This feeling accompanied me through some of the darkest moments of my life. The peace I was able to create under some very painful circumstances was extraordinary.

I was lucky to find something that ultimately became a universal truth for me. Did I make it up? Yes, of course I did. What I would like to suggest to those who are searching for something to hang on to is this: You have permission to create any belief system that offers you comfort. It does not take away from or impose itself upon the beliefs of another. It is yours and yours alone. I am sure that some would feel I am out of my mind for the way I think. But perhaps that is exactly what we need, to be out of our minds, so that we can truly be in our hearts and souls.

———

I WAS GRATEFUL to have God by my side. I was about to start a journey I was ill prepared for, and it was comforting to know that I would not have to do it alone—I had my constant companion in my heart and soul. Finding a sense of peace within myself and feeling supported unconditionally allowed me to embark on a brand-new adventure with the sense of having my hand held. It gave me the strength to forge into the unknown with grace and with ease. There was no guarantee that whatever I was willing to do or try would ensure I'd live long enough to see my girls grow up, but I was not discouraged. The goal of being there for my daughters was my initial driving force. Eventually I picked up the reigns and chose life for myself. I am not sure when that transition happened; I only know that it did.

Finding myself as a result of this saga was an unexpected gift, for I never realized at the time that I had gone missing. I'd always known I was a good mother, wife, sister, daughter, and friend, but I wondered: Without those roles, who was I, really? Who was this woman named Susan Wener, and what was she willing to do to keep herself alive? I could fight for my family in a heartbeat, but could I really learn to fight for myself? I hated fighting. I spent my entire life as a peacekeeper. Everybody came to me with their problems, and I made time for them all, even when it took away from what I needed to do for myself. I wondered if I would be able to learn how to take care of my own needs before the needs of those around me. Could I do that and not care about how I was perceived? (That may have been part of the problem with my mother-in-law. I so badly wanted her to like and think well of me. Instead of finding my voice and speaking my truth, I lost myself in an illusion of what I thought a mother-and-daughter-in-law relationship should be. Could I change without losing the essence of me in the process?)

Over the many years that followed, I learned the difference between selfishness and self-preservation. Being selfish means doing something for yourself even though it might harm another. Self-preservation, however, means doing whatever is necessary to keep yourself healthy and strong, without causing harm to another (at least not intentionally). I had to learn the difference between what was mine to fix and what belonged to someone else. No matter how difficult it was initially, I came to understand that I could not fix anyone else. Offering guidance and compassion was fine, but not if it came at the price of depleting my own energy resources. I needed to develop boundaries of steel. Inside those boundaries I had to keep everything I required for survival; anything that might drain me had to stay outside. This was not going to be an easy task.

Wow! And I thought all I was going to have to deal with was cancer! I was being thrown into self-actualization long before I was ready. I used to think that the universe gave us little taps on the shoulder when things weren't working well, to help direct us toward a better path. Had I been so unobservant that the gentle tap on the shoulder had turned into a sledgehammer over my head? Had the previous surgeries not been enough? I couldn't seem to get the phrase, "ultimate failure of the body's immune system" out of my head: the *ultimate* failure. Well, my mother always told me that if I was going to do something, I should do it well.

Enough of that: enough of going backwards. I decided I would explore options in both the traditional and nontraditional worlds on my road toward healing. I did not want to be judged for my choices. I wanted to be supported with kindness and compassion. Slowly but surely, I was creating a plan for myself. It felt good to have something to hold on to.

My main objective was to live long enough to ensure that my daughters grew into strong and independent women. I so badly wanted them to love themselves and realize their worth. I wanted them to see themselves just as I saw them. They would probably never really understand the depths of my love for them until they had children of their own. I thought they were loving, sensitive, and incredible young girls. I was so proud to be their mother.

All right, I had created my own concept of God. That was a good start. And now I had an objective, but what next?

All I knew was that I needed to live. I believed with all my heart that I wasn't done yet. As much as I loved my husband, I knew he would be fine. I remembered telling him that if I died, I wanted him to be happy and have someone to share his life with. The only thing I insisted on was that he was not allowed to date anyone who brought him shivah casseroles. Shivah, in the Jewish religion, is when you sit in mourning for seven days after an immediate family member is buried. Traditionally, relatives, friends, and neighbors prepare the mourners' food. Jon loves to eat, and I wasn't having someone win his heart through his stomach. I thought this was hysterical and burst out laughing after I said it. He, unfortunately, did not seem to share my sense of humor.

So here I was, ready to embark on a journey anywhere away from the drama I was presently living. To this day, I am still in awe of my family's capacity to simply live their lives. How seamless it appeared to be for them. It's not as though I wanted them to stay home and suffer, but their ability to adapt forced me to accept the fact that their lives would go on with or without me. I was left with lots of time on my hands. I was forced to redefine my role as wife and mother. Whether I liked it or not, it was time to face myself. I decided that since my whole world felt a bit out of control, I needed structure.

I remember sitting down with pen in hand, trying to write a list of all the things and people that made me feel good and contributed to the quality of my life. I also made a list of all those who did not. I then gave myself permission (because who could argue with a poor cancer patient, after all) to get rid of or change all that seemed to be disharmonious in my life. If I didn't like someone (even if they were a family member), I didn't have to be with them. Believe me, it was not as easy as it sounds. I was often riddled with guilt. (I have learned since then that guilt is such a useless emotion. Remorse forces us to make amends, but guilt just eats us up alive.) If there was an event that I didn't want to go to, I didn't even have to make up an excuse. I simply didn't go. Yeah! Cancer was proving to have some secondary gains after all. For the first time in my life, I allowed myself to do or not do whatever I wanted. I moved with my reptilian brain away from danger and toward harmony. What the hell had taken me so long? Did I really need this disease to learn how to just say no? Had I previously been a mere pawn at everyone's beck and call? Never again, I determined.

Years later, Jon asked me, when we were having a bit of a tiff, "Whatever happened to that sweet little girl I married?" I replied, "She's dead, and the strong woman you never realized you wanted has taken her place. If you don't like it, too bad, because she's the one who is staying!" Perhaps the words came out a little harsher than they needed to, but I didn't care. It is difficult when one person in a family decides to make drastic changes. It has a domino effect and upsets the equilibrium of the entire family. Ultimately, my transformation was really good for my family, and my husband grew to love the strong and independent woman I was becoming. As I learned to take care of my own needs, my family in turn learned to take care of theirs. The difference was that they didn't have to get sick in order to get permission to take care of themselves.

(5)

THE WELLNESS PUZZLE

PHYSICALLY I WAS recovering nicely. Three weeks after surgery, I had no residual physical effects. We are far more than just physical beings, however, and I knew that the emotional and psychological consequences of the illness would follow in due course. "One thing at a time," I told myself. It still did not take much to overwhelm me. What I needed was guidance to help me with the steps ahead.

After I had my spine fused when I was thirty-two, my doctor advised me not to lift and turn patients the way I had done before. I stopped working in palliative care at the Royal Victoria Hospital and began volunteering at the Jewish General Hospital for Hope & Cope, a nonprofit organization founded in 1981 by Sheila Kussner. She had lost her leg to cancer as a teenager and realized how few services were available to provide information and advice to cancer patients. She made it her mission to do just that. Today, Hope & Cope is renowned for its excellence not only in patient care but in teaching and research as well. Sheila always understood that the physical impact of cancer is only one aspect patients need to address. She and her organization help confront the emotional and spiritual aspects of cancer by offering comprehensive tools and programs to patients and family members affected by this disease. With my training in palliative care, Sheila and I started a team of volunteers who would visit and help those who were dying.

It was now time for me to see how I might best use this incredible resource. I turned to Jean Remmer, one of the women who worked at Hope & Cope. There was little advice or direction offered back then with regards to alternative medicine. What existed, however, was a lot of empathy, attention, and respect. Everyone who worked in the organization had dealt with cancer on a personal level, and they were able to offer the wisdom and support only those who had walked the journey could offer. Jean became my sounding board and my safe place. To this day, I am grateful to her and to Sheila for creating an organization dedicated to improving the lives of so many. I talked to them about chemotherapy before I started it. The plan was for me to have six months of chemotherapy. It would be administered five days in a row, with twenty-one days between cycles. I was scared, and they were able to reassure me that many patients had survived it. They promised that they would be there to support me should I need it.

I tried to appear as calm as possible the morning I left for my first chemo session, but I was terrified and shaking inside. Jon closed his eyes when the procedure was about to start. He is quite squeamish when it comes to medical stuff (I used to watch operations on television and he would walk out of the room). As soon as the needle entered my vein, I threw up. "Anticipatory nausea," the nurses told me. "Great," I thought, "so much for my attempts to keep it together!" What a way to start.

The treatments on Monday and Tuesday were not too bad. By the time Wednesday rolled around, I was sick. It was not easy getting me to the hospital for the rest of the treatments, but I persevered. I tried to drug myself and sleep as best I could. My oncologist advised that I would be tired and need lots of rest the second week. Not me! Knowing that I had twenty-one days free of treatment gave me the boost I needed to manage well, tending to my family's needs. I pretended that my real life existed between treatments. I rarely complained to Jon or the girls and simply did my best to function and appear normal to the outside world. My inside world, however, felt anything but normal.

Things changed midway through my fifth cycle. I started to feel very strange. It was early evening and I tried to reach Jon, who was away in Ottawa on a business trip. There was a terrible ice storm that day, and all the airplanes in and out of Montreal had been cancelled. We finally connected after a couple hours. He told me to try to relax and that if I needed him, he would rent a car and drive home. I thought I was having an anxiety attack and took a bath to calm down. Nothing worked, and I was getting myself more and more worked up and upset.

I called my friend Anita, who came right over. She took one look at me and knew that something was wrong. My body was contorted, my neck twisted, and I was having serious trouble breathing. She called Alex, my oncologist, and described the symptoms. He was at the hospital, which was not far from my house. He jumped into his truck (which could get through the ice) and drove over. It took him a minute to realize that this was not anxiety. I was having a severe allergic reaction to one of the medications given to me during chemotherapy. My breathing passages were shutting down.

My kids were scared. I will never forget the look of horror on their faces as Alex carried me over his shoulder and down the stairs to take me to the hospital. They were terrified and clinging to one another, tears pouring down their faces. Anita stayed at the house to keep things under control, and the doctor promised to call as soon as he had some news. In the meantime, my husband had a colleague drive him home from Ottawa. He was too nervous to drive himself. It was a nightmare for all of us.

Carol-Ann had been my angel, and Alex quickly became my knight in shining armor. I barely knew this man other than seeing him at the hospital. I could hardly believe that he was so attentive to a virtual stranger. People complain all the time about the quality of care they receive. Not me. There were very few glitches along my journey, and for that I am eternally grateful. The kindness of my doctors truly aided my journey toward recovery. I felt as though they were part of my team, part of what I liked to call my wellness puzzle. They did not just dispense a service. I felt special. I felt taken care of. And I will never forget their role in my life. I am sure that even today, so many years later, had Alex remained in Montreal, he would still be an integral part of my life, as Carol-Ann is.

When I went to sleep that night, I lay there wondering why, if I had a ninety-five percent chance of disease-free living, did I find myself crying at the drop of a hat? I would be driving the car and a song on the radio could produce enough tears to force me off the road. As much as I hated the chemotherapy, to be told that my body could no longer tolerate it left me terrified. I had not even finished five out of the six cycles. Would it have all been for naught, I wondered? I asked Alex if he would consider hospitalizing me for the last five-day cycle, just so that I could finish the protocol. He refused. He told me that even if I were his wife or mother, he would have to say no.

When the body says no, it really means no. What was I to do now? I had originally thought that I would simply be able to get on with my life when I finished chemotherapy. What I found instead was that I would fall apart if someone just looked at me the wrong way. I was even more vulnerable than before. For the first time in my life, this strong, capable woman actually felt fragile. It didn't matter how many previous surgeries I had sailed through. This was a different story. This was cancer, the "Big C." I did not know the outcome. I could not be certain I would survive it.

When I was twenty-seven years old, Jon, Jacqueline, Kassy, and I went to Maine for a holiday (Ali had not yet been born). As we walked along the Marginal Way, a street filled with shops and restaurants, we stopped to see a palm reader. Jon thought I was nuts, but I thought it would be fun. She looked at the palms of Jon and the girls and said that they loved the water and that they each had strong personalities. I thought, "How silly, of course they love the water; that is why we chose this holiday."

Then it was my turn. When she looked at my palm, she turned as white as a ghost. "You will have a life filled with pain, suffering, and illness," she said. "You will probably die young." I picked up the kids and ran out of there. Her words traumatized me for more than six months. How could she tell me that? Did she really know what the future had in store for me?

Now, as I pondered her words nine years later, I wondered if her prophecy would be proven correct. Would I ever get to see my girls grow up? All the doctors could offer me as reassurance were routine checkups. "Get on with your life and you will be fine," they told me. How can anyone say that? Did they really believe it themselves? What did that even mean? Did they expect me to simply close the book and pretend that the illness never happened? There was no way I was going to hang around waiting to see if the cancer might come back. As strange as it may sound, I felt protected while undergoing chemotherapy. I know that the side effects of nausea, diarrhea, fatigue, and hair loss were not exactly a picnic, but I believed that they demonstrated that the drugs were indeed working. Now that it was over, I was on my own. I needed to find something to fill the space between the end of treatment and optimal health. I needed to get into gear immediately and start moving forward. I needed to discover more components of my own wellness puzzle, for my peace of mind as well as my sanity. Each piece had to be something meaningful to me. I knew God was definitely one. Traditional medicine was another. In the years ahead, I would discover many aspects, physically, spiritually, and emotionally, that would make my puzzle complete. I would shift and change the pieces when needed, which gave me a kind of structural freedom that worked well with my personality.

————

· the wellness puzzle ·

I LIKE TO look at health and well-being as a puzzle. Each piece of the puzzle represents something important to the patient. Although the components of everyone's puzzle are different, as health care providers, we need to respect what is important to our patients if we want to truly help them through a very difficult time. Although we may not always agree with their choices, this mutual respect keeps the pathways of communication open. No one can ever guarantee any outcome. What we can guarantee, however, is that we will do our best to look at the individual needs of the patient and try to tailor a program that suits them. This makes living so much easier for both health care provider and patient.

In many cases, medicine is not linear. Because everyone is different, we will respond differently to whatever treatment program we may choose. The success of any treatment protocol can be affected by our state of physical, emotional, and spiritual health, as well as our thoughts and beliefs. So we must attend to each of these aspects, creating the optimal internal environment for getting the results we want from any treatment we may choose.

———

One of the most revolutionary ideas in the New Age movement (a movement centered on incorporating alternative and complementary practices as part of whole person care) is that of personal responsibility. Most people hate this concept because it puts the onus for action on them. It pushes them to partner in their own health care process. I do not believe that doctors cure patients. They simply offer the very best of their craft, be it surgical, medical, or psychological. It is vital that patients understand that it is their responsibility to create an optimal internal environment so that whatever treatment course they may choose will have the best chance of being effective. This idea of responsibility can be both daunting and empowering. On one hand, self-blame when something does not work is not helpful. On the other hand, we don't need to wait to begin taking care of ourselves. This gives us permission to participate in our healing process, long before formal treatment begins. It makes us feel as though we are actually helping ourselves, rather than sitting around waiting to see how the cards may fall.

I figured that we basically do three things to maintain our health:

1. We put food in our mouths.
2. We exercise our bodies.
3. We put thought in our minds.

I was on a mission to improve all three. As well as I thought I had been doing on these fronts, I must have been looking through rose-colored glasses. Much to my family's chagrin, I started with what I thought was the easiest of the three: food. There was so much to read on the subject, and every train of thought had some validity to it. After much deliberation, I decided to become not just a vegetarian but a vegan. Forget the easy road; I was determined that no animal product or by-product would touch my lips. Both my daughter Kassy and my sister were already vegetarians. Kassy made the decision by age eleven, and Linda changed her eating habits to help reme-diate some health issues she was dealing with. They had no trouble eating this way, so I figured that I would try it, too.

One of the very frustrating things for someone after a diag-nosis of cancer is the idea of "What now?" Do we simply wait until doctors find something wrong with us and then treat it, or can we fill in that gap ourselves? I liked the idea of doing some-thing for myself. I couldn't stand the wait-and-see game. Food is an essential component to health and well-being. It provides us with the vital energy we need to make it through the day. It helps to remind us that we can still feel good and enjoy life even after a diagnosis of cancer. Food, in some ways, was easy to deal with. No one could force me to eat or drink what I didn't want to. Although cancer is said to be "the body out of control," it felt empowering to be in control of something again. I had God, I had traditional medicine, I had an objective (helping my kids find their strengths), and now I also had food. I was finding the pieces in my puzzle.

I wore vegetarianism on my shoulder like a badge. I felt that I was part of an exclusive club. Not only did everyone I meet find out by the end of the conversation that I had had cancer, but they also knew that I was a vegetarian. It was almost as though I was trying to convince myself on a regular basis that this was actually good for me. I am by nature a private person, and this was very strange behavior. I found myself talking nonstop with anyone who would listen. Clearly I had a strong need to be heard. It was as though everyone I met became my sounding board. I suppose that by not wanting to rock the boat, and by allowing a sick relationship with my mother-in-law to continue far too long, I had stuffed my voice deep down inside myself for a very long time. It was my turn to be heard, even if it was inappropriate at times.

I suffered terribly from my food choices. Just because we decide to change our lifestyle, that doesn't mean the education to make good choices immediately becomes available. I was not very good at combining foods, and I suffered from protein deprivation. Living off bread, beans, vegetables, and fruit did not seem to do the trick. I longed for that scrambled egg my mom used to make me when I felt sick. I found myself salivating for the hot dogs my kids ate behind my back when they thought I wasn't looking. I was miserable, my family was miserable, and my husband gained at least twenty pounds looking for food in all the wrong places. I didn't only watch what I ate; I also watched what everyone else ate. I was on a mission and became a complete pain in the ass. I became the extremist to the extreme. No one wanted to bring their friends home for dinner; in fact, no one even wanted dinner!

Today, I deprive myself of nothing. When I want a treat, I have it and enjoy it completely. I figure that if it makes me feel that good, it must therefore be good for me. I remind myself that a treat is special because it only occurs once in a while. I am no longer rigid with my diet, but I am a conscious eater, which I think is important. I found that I could eat one cookie or a few potato chips and all hell did not break loose. I could have whatever I wanted, and therefore nothing needed to be hoarded. I felt continuously satisfied. I began to realize that it is only when we deny ourselves that cravings take on a life of their own. I am not suggesting we live on junk food. I am talking about a diet of real food, including fruits, vegetables, nuts, grains and seeds, meat, fish, poultry, and dairy products. I always believed that only twenty percent of our plates should be animal products. The best way to go, I think, is to fill the remaining eighty percent with fruits and vegetables, nuts, grains, and seeds. This was easy for me to follow because it was how my mom fed us at home. Dr. Richard Béliveau, an authority in cancer research, confirms this approach. He holds the Chair in Cancer Prevention and Treatment at the University of Quebec at Montreal. In his book *Foods That Fight Cancer*, he explains some of the research showing which foods may be of benefit in both preventing and overcoming cancer. Further research demonstrates the correlation between diet and how we feel physically, mentally, and spiritually.

I started really listening to my body and determined that it was my best teacher. Eating healthfully helped me to feel balanced. Listening to the needs of my body (with the understanding that those needs change on a regular basis), instead of restricting myself, became the answer for me.

Am I perfect? Absolutely not! Do I like that occasional hot dog all-dressed? Oh, yes! The fact that I might have one only a few times a year is what makes it so special. What you do on a regular basis always overshadows what you do occasionally. My family was so relieved by my changed attitude toward food that everyone rejoined me at the dinner table. Eating became fun once again. We laughed and talked freely when we were together. I was more relaxed, and so was everyone else.

———

· *diet* ·

THERE IS SO much written today about health and nutrition that I sometimes think there are more theories out there than the people pushing them. Everyone has an opinion on the subject. Eat this, don't eat that; drink this, don't drink that; raw food versus cooked food; contractive foods verses expansive foods. I think that all this focus can sometimes make people crazy, especially when charismatic individuals speak passionately about what they believe to be true.

I am not going to agree or disagree with any of these theories. Whatever works for you is fine. What I will say, however, is that when we are ill and we feel we have somehow lost control of our body, food may be one of the few things we have some power over. That in itself is vital to our well-being. When our whole world is falling apart, we need to feel that we are somehow helping ourselves. Food can do far more than merely nourish a body. It can also help soothe the soul. As Marc David says in his book

Nourishing Wisdom, "the attitude with which we eat is sometimes just as important as what we eat."

———

Exercise had never been difficult for me to incorporate into my life. I was always very physical and preferred walking and playing sports to spending hours in the gym. When I was a little girl, my mother used to take my siblings and me on long walks in the country. She was so fast that my little legs could barely keep up with her. I in turn spent hours walking with my children and had them out of their strollers long before their third birthdays. It was important to me that they become strong enough to enjoy life fully. Being active has always been an integral part of our lives.

After spinal surgery, my doctor advised me to stretch daily, keep limber, and maintain my weight. I found this very easy to do, and it became as routine as brushing my teeth. The change I made after colon cancer was to ensure that I never exhausted myself. I had always loved the feeling of being totally spent after dancing—I worked so hard in my practices that I looked as though I had just come out of the shower, soaked in sweat from head to toe. But I believed that my body had been traumatized by the surgery and especially by the chemotherapy. What it seemed to require now was to be treated with gentle loving-kindness. That translated into resting before I tired and going about my life with a bit less intensity. It was my hope that these small changes would start to supplement my depleted energy.

Food and exercise were pretty easy for me to get a handle on. Changing the thoughts in my mind, however, was a whole different kettle of fish. I had become fearful, and this concern over my health was growing into a preoccupation. Before I got sick, I thought I knew my body. What I realized instead was that I had actually abused it. Some people think that dancers are amazing with their bodies and that they have the capacity to hear what each muscle and tendon has to say. I did not listen to my body's messages. Even when it hurt, I pushed through the pain. "No pain, no gain" was what I recall my instructors telling me. I did not know any better. I listened to my teachers and believed in their expertise. The thing I did learn from dance, however, was discipline. Whatever I set my mind to, I accomplished. Perhaps this was the lesson I needed to remember as I headed into uncharted waters.

(6)

THE MIND AS
A POWER TOOL

ALTHOUGH MY FUTURE looked bright from a medical perspective, I would say that for a good year following surgery I was still very sensitive. I hated hearing people say, "Don't worry, everything will be fine." They thought they were being kind. I thought they were being foolish. "Don't worry"—what a joke. By nature, I am an optimistic person. But my Pollyanna nature was definitely being tested. My goal became to stay alive long enough to see my kids graduate from high school.

I started meeting with a doctor who taught me creative visualization. Even as a little girl, I had a bold and vivid imagination. I was powerfully drawn to the idea of creating an inner world that made me feel better. Today there is so much written on the science of neuroplasticity. It shows us that the brain is not static and has the potential to actually change during the course of our lifetime. All it needs is training and practice. Visualization was a way for me to tap into that source of limitless potential. The best part was that I did not have to go anywhere to access it. It exists inside me.

I ended up studying creative visualization for more than two years. When I decided to start teaching others what had become so helpful to me, my mentor became my first client. I had always known that, on some level, our minds could be our best friend or our worst enemy. My challenge became how to use my mind effectively. I watched myself soar through many surgeries, using my mind as an ally. But I also watched myself spiral into a black hole, wondering if I would live or die after a diagnosis of cancer.

―――

· *creative visualization* ·

CREATIVE VISUALIZATION IS a mental technique. It is a tool that can help us move beyond perceived limitations. We can learn to use our imaginations to help us achieve our desired goals.

For example, sports psychologists use it to teach professional skiers to foresee every bump and turn on the hill as they practice for their races. As children, we read about how the "little engine that could" made it up the mountain against seemingly impossible odds. We encourage our children to continue facing their challenges, even when they might feel like giving up. We try to get them to see themselves as successful. We also endeavor to help our partners to see "the bigger picture." We daydream about falling in love. At a romantic movie, we might even create a sexual fantasy (that is one way to prove that a mind-body connection definitely exists!).

Creative visualization is a form of wishful thinking. We can train ourselves to use it on a daily basis to help produce positive changes in our lives. We need to learn how to use our minds with intention.

―――

I decided that I needed to use my mind in the same way I would use a power tool, to help me forge a path toward health and well-being. Now, don't get me wrong, just because you wish for something doesn't mean you automatically get it. Creating the picture, fueling it with passion and desire, encourages you to take the necessary steps to reach your goal. I often hear people say, "That's wishful thinking," as if it's a bad thing. It is not. Wishful thinking is what keeps us alive. It is what gives us hope for a better tomorrow.

· ·

· *the placebo effect* ·

MANY OF US have heard of the term "placebo effect." A placebo is a medically ineffectual treatment, such as a sugar pill. Very often, a patient who is given a placebo will still experience either a perceived or actual improvement of whatever medical condition they are dealing with. The placebo effect is scientifically well documented. We know placebos work about twenty percent of the time. Our minds are mysterious and are capable of creating the reaction we expect. Although the results may not be long-lasting for everyone, the understanding that our beliefs have the ability to influence our physiology is not only incredible but empowering as well. Imagine adding a twenty percent potential success rate to any chosen treatment program. Is that just wishful thinking?

I believe that we can train ourselves to use the placebo effect on purpose. Would you prefer to see chemotherapy as a poison harming you or as a magic elixir knowing exactly where it needs to go to get to those cancer cells? Would you ever take a headache pill if you didn't believe that it knew where to go to relieve the headache? Of course not. I have always understood that our belief systems help create our reality. The power the mind can have over the body is real. Our beliefs are the very basic foundations of our lives. If we believe we are doing something good for us, then that belief in itself can often help us do whatever may be necessary to reach that perceived reality. If we are unable to reach our goal, however, the quality of our lives in our attempt to get there will still be greatly enhanced. For me, living a life where no hope exists is not living!

———

I remember an Orthodox Jewish man asking to meet me privately to discuss the work I was doing with his wife. He begged me to get his wife to try harder to believe that she could get better. She had a very painful kind of bone cancer and was struggling to make it through each day. I had seen her as a private client for about six months and did my best to help her discover the stress management tools that worked best for her. I asked him what would happen if her body was just too tired to fight any longer. He sadly lowered his eyes and said that he would then lose his best friend.

Hope, faith, and belief make living easier, no matter what we may have to face. Healing, however, sometimes comes with acceptance, even if that means acceptance of death. Sometimes the body is just too exhausted to support life. Accepting death is not a failure or a lack of hope. Perhaps it is simply a hope for a better tomorrow. We may not understand what awaits us at the end of our lives, but since none of us know for certain what is on the other side, I would like to believe that it is filled with the magic of possibility. Having that little bit of hope is often enough to make living each day just a little bit easier.

——

· *hope* ·

WIKIPEDIA DEFINES HOPE as the "state which promotes the desire of positive outcomes related to events and circumstances in one's life." Viktor Frankl was an Austrian psychiatrist who wrote about the horrors of the Holocaust in his book *Man's Search for Meaning.* He felt that without hope, the human race would not have survived. Hope gives us something to hang on to.

Dr. Herbert Benson says that in the absence of certainty, there is nothing wrong with hope. I laugh when doctors mock the various coping strategies we may use when we are in crisis. Don't they understand that the very concept of "wishful thinking" ("the attribution of reality to what one wishes to be true or the tenuous justification of what one wants to believe," according to *Webster's*) is often the main ingredient keeping us alive? The hope that tomorrow will be better, the hope of making it to a planned event, the hope of hearing good news, could be that magic elixir that heals the soul.

——

Everyone will face difficulties and challenges in their lifetime. Our capacity to pick ourselves up, dust ourselves off, and start again blows me away. Hope and optimism are two of the many tools I carry with me everywhere I go. I have many other components that fill my own wellness puzzle. Some of them are as simple as friend and family time, whereas others are more complex, including different systems of medicine, such as homeopathy or Chinese medical practices. The specifics of each person's puzzle are not important. They are different for every one of us and often change throughout our lives. What is important is that we recognize and find those things that fill us and make us feel good. By choosing to incorporate them into our lives, we have a better chance of coping well during the difficult times.

On December 11, 1996, I spoke at a conference entitled "Alternative Medicine—Fact or Fancy," held at the Montreal Children's Hospital. I only realized once the conference ended that its objective was to discredit various forms of alternative medicine (Quebec had little tolerance in general for alternative medicine back in the nineties). Thank goodness I did not know this beforehand, as I am not sure I would have been able to get up and speak. I started by explaining the potential benefits of visualization. I talked about teaching cancer patients how to create a private sanctuary for themselves. It would be a place where they could go and imagine themselves cancer-free, healthy, and enjoying life fully.

One doctor raised his hand and said, "Susan Wener, you are full of shit! How dare you tell someone filled with tumors to imagine themselves cancer-free? You are being irrational and unethical. What you are actually doing is creating false hope."

It was funny to see my husband's face in the audience. His mouth dropped open and fire filled his eyes. He was aghast that someone would speak to me like that. He had gone to summer camp with this doctor, but for a moment I thought he might leap from his chair and strangle him. We protect the ones we love, and I was grateful to have him there supporting me.

What most people don't know about me is that I love to be challenged. This was right up my alley. I asked the doctor to look at what I was saying from a business perspective. If he were going to create a new business, would he want to surround himself with people who showed him how it could work, or with those who told him how it might fail? Whereas the latter is very important and must also be addressed, it is the former that drives passion and propels us toward our goal. We need to encourage ourselves to keep pushing forward in order to overcome obstacles. Step by step is the only way I know how to continuously move forward without losing sight of my projected goal. I told him that cancer patients rarely forget that they are sick. What they need are distractions. They are looking for anything that might take them away from what is painful (either physically or psychologically). If they can find a quiet place in their minds, where they can disappear, even for a few moments, and feel healthy, well, and strong, is that really such a bad thing?

We need to remember that we are not just treating a disease. We are treating people living with a disease. That fact is difficult enough to remember for those of us who are enduring cancer. Any respite from pain and suffering is welcome. We have the ability to create that respite within ourselves by using our minds. This way of thinking simply makes living easier. Perhaps that is what hope, belief, and wishful thinking are supposed to do. They offer us moments of relief. Believe me, the journey through cancer is hellish enough. If we can find a way to make living through it easier, then I am all for it.

· *private sanctuary* ·

Take my hand and help me run
To that place of freedom
To that place of sun.
I need to go where the monsters aren't
To the sanity of safety
To the calmness of heart
To taste the sweetness
The nectar of hope
The words that soothe
The thoughts that help me cope
To see myself as I yearn to be
The perfection of all the potential in me.
I bathe and soak in the quiet and peace;
It is here I wish for a lifetime lease.
I go and visit in the quiet of night
That place of freedom that is my right.

I received a standing ovation from the other doctors in the auditorium for my response. After asking them to sit back down, I explained that this was not a matter of my being right or the doctor who confronted me being wrong. This was a matter of education. Thinking differently often requires explanation. We cannot possibly know everything. That is why we often look to others for guidance. We need to learn how to use everything available to us in order to live as best we can, irrespective of what we may have to face.

I found out later that the doctor who challenged me at the conference had been frustrated when one of his young patients turned to a form of alternative medicine and died in the process. I would never encourage anyone to give up one form of medicine for another unless they were certain that the one they abandoned was of no benefit to them. However, I urge everyone, whether sick or well, to look around at all the options that may be available to them and use them to the best of their advantage.

What works for some may not work for others. That does not make the treatments good or bad. It means that each one of us has unique needs, and we must hunt until we find the ones that work best for us. Imagery and visualization can be learned easily. We don't even realize that we use these techniques effortlessly every day. Different forms of self-hypnosis are another approach that can be helpful to some. Libraries, bookstores, and resource centers are full of books on these subjects. The techniques are simple enough that everybody can learn them quickly. Our job is to learn how to use them with a purpose in mind.

People die every day from cancer. All our efforts may not lead us to the cure we're seeking. How we deal with that realization may greatly impact whatever time we do have left on this earth. Our minds may be our best ally to help us hope and cope as we journey through life's ups and downs. Even if our life is not extended, its quality can be vastly improved. Faith, belief, and wishful thinking are sometimes all that is needed to keep us moving forward, right until the end, with grace and with ease.

After one of my visualization training sessions, I remember talking to my daughters about what I was learning. They asked me how I saw my future. I told them that although I could not promise them that I would never get sick again, I could promise them that I wasn't done living yet. I was beginning to create an inner self-confidence that I had never had before. When I graduated from university, I was worried that I would not get a teaching job. Would I be good enough? Would anybody want me? I was quite young (just twenty-two years old) and lacked self-confidence. I think part of me chose to become pregnant before I graduated so that I wouldn't have to face the possibility of rejection. I was perfectly fine with this, since it was in alignment with my desire to become a mother. However, I was very surprised when I received eight offers to teach!

Fear and negative thinking seemed to have a strong hold on me back then. Although the expression "negative thinking" seems to have become an acceptable term for describing unwelcome thoughts, I dislike its implications. It makes you feel that you are somehow to blame for the thoughts that cross your path. Part of being human is experiencing all kinds of thoughts—the good, the bad, the ugly, and the sad. Often, these thoughts are fleeting. To feel that we are somehow hurting ourselves by thinking them is not helpful, especially at a time when we are already vulnerable. It is all right to think and feel everything.

My clients often ask me why it feels so much easier to sink into a black hole than to climb out of one. So I simply throw a pencil up in the air and ask them to notice how gravity has a way of pulling everything downward. It is always harder to push uphill against a force of nature. It is amazing, though, how relieved they feel when I tell them that it is all right to visit that black and bleak place. "Visit, just don't take up residence there!" I say.

They feel as though these few words I have given them are a gift. We all need to accept that it is all right to sometimes feel miserable and fall apart. To deny the thoughts and feelings that may not be pretty is to deny a part of ourselves. Our feelings are how we differ not only from the animal in the wild but from one another. There is nothing wrong with any of them, and all are appropriate in different circumstances.

Humans also differ from the wild animal in the sense that we have "a thinking brain." But sometimes I think that our cerebral cortex, the thinking and planning part of our brain, gets in our way. We often overthink situations, are highly critical of ourselves, and at times become so confused that we may even develop paralysis from analysis! Instead of moving forward, we just swim around in circles, festering in our experience of the moment.

Problems can arise based on how long we choose to stay in that dark place or whether we are able to emerge from it on our own. My daughter Kassy used to get angry with me when I tried to encourage her to change her thinking. She needed to wallow in her discomfort and self-pity until she was good and ready to make the shift herself. No matter how difficult it was for me to watch her misery, I learned to step back and allow her to be who she needed to be. When she finally made the shift, it was as though an entirely different perspective opened up for her. It was wonderful to see. She reminded me not to try to rush the river, and to allow people the time they need to process their issues.

ONCE I FINISHED my creative visualization training, I announced that I wanted to use it to teach other people. I had graduated from university as a teacher, and it was now time to open up a practice and share what I had learned from my training. Visualization made me feel calm and in better control of my thoughts and feelings. It was kind of like a blissful form of meditation, but instead of trying to think about nothing, my mind became filled with all the wonderful thoughts and feelings that made me happy and peaceful. My soul began to feel more settled.

I was amazed by how many clients started to come. Everyone had something in common: they were all hungry and desperate to feel good. It really doesn't matter how different our stories are; we all appear to have similar basic needs. Feeling good happens to be one of them.

Part of my job became guiding my clients toward finding the resources that helped them to feel better. I came across a poem by Steven Javan Jones that had a lot of impact on me. "We are born into the world," it begins, "like a blank canvas." Everyone we meet, the poem continues, "Takes up the brush / And makes his mark / Upon our surface." Ultimately, though, we have to take responsibility for painting our own canvas:

> But we must realize there comes a day
> That we must take up the brush
> And finish the work.
> For only we can determine
> If we are to be
> Just another painting
> Or a masterpiece.

We must pick up the brush. I realized that others may guide or influence us, but we are the ones who actually have to do the work. My aunt once said she would prefer to take a pill rather than do any work herself. She felt that the latter was just too difficult for her. "Illness is hard enough," she said. "Why should I have to put so much effort into getting better if there are different options out there?" I found this sentiment very interesting. My aunt's words made me realize that we are not taught how to pick up that brush when we are ill. We are expected to rely on the medical expertise available to us. Our doctors don't have time to offer the psychological and emotional counsel we need when we are diagnosed with a life-threatening illness. They are far too busy trying to save our lives. When I thought about my aunt's words, I realized how many people would rather take "the pill" than change their lives. Change your diet or take a pill? It is much harder to make changes than it is to swallow a simple tablet. It means you are accountable.

I once asked my dad to give up smoked meat sandwiches and hot dogs because he always got heartburn after eating them. He told me that he would rather take an antacid pill than give them up because they truly made him happy. We so badly want to feel good that we are willing to be soothed by whatever gives us even temporary pleasure. Sometimes the price we pay for that moment of pleasure can be incredibly high.

That was the feeling I had when I was first diagnosed with cancer. "Take care of me, hold my hand, do whatever you have to do to make me better. I'm in." Perhaps when we are first told we are sick, we are not capable of doing the work ourselves. We require all of our energy just to keep ourselves glued together. But in time, unless we decide to pick up the brush ourselves, we might go only where the wind blows us. For me, "the work" gave me freedom. My outcome wasn't going to be solely determined by anyone else (as I had decided when I made my partnership with God).

If I was going to change old patterns that were not serving me well, I needed to deal with confrontation head on. Silencing myself and swallowing my pain contributed to my suffering. Things had to change. I had held my tongue long enough. I had stuffed enough frustration into my gut to last a lifetime. The pattern of saying nothing was not working for me any longer. I needed to break free from my cocoon and learn to stand up for myself with strength, not with anger or frustration. It was time. There was no way I was going to be just another painting. I was going to become a masterpiece! Move over, Picasso, here comes Susan!

I realized that I had lots of work to do. It was time to go back to school.

(7)

BACK TO SCHOOL

I JOINED THE Natural Health Consultants Institute, a non-profit school of holistic health care founded in 1991 by Nancy Hamilton. I enrolled in the second year of the school's existence, and as a new institution, it still had a lot of cobwebs to be cleared out. I needed to learn and explore the correlation between body, mind, spirit, and soul. It was important for me to expand beyond traditional medicine and look at other factors that contribute to sickness, healing, and well-being.

At that time, the program was a three-year commitment. It was so different from anything I had ever been exposed to, and I wondered initially if I had been teleported onto Mars. I soon discovered, however, that I could keep my feet on the ground, become discerning, and still accomplish my goal of learning about integrative health. One of the courses I took was about personal development. It helped me find out a lot about myself and encouraged me to work through some personal limitations I had self imposed (such as not being sure I could ever again trust my body to be perfectly healthy).

One of the exercises we did regularly was free-flow writing. That meant picking a topic (for me that was easy: cancer, fear, health, death, safety, sanity) and writing about it for fifteen to twenty minutes straight without ever lifting the pen off the paper or reviewing what we had written. Spelling and grammar didn't count, and since there was no judgment on our writing, we could not get it wrong. This kind of writing gets the creative juices flowing and can be very revealing. It seems to tap into the subconscious mind. Many therapists use this as a tool to help themselves and others when dealing with complex or difficult situations. I loved it. I could write about anything. I simply started to write, and to this day I continue to practice free-flow writing and encourage my clients to do it as well. It helps me manage daily stress. It allows me to find my voice in a safe way, without worrying that I might be hurting anyone.

There was a whole new world out there for me to discover. My eyes were beginning to open. I wondered how I would extract what I needed from the multitude of options that existed. I was a neophyte in school, with no idea how to process all the information I was being exposed to. It was a lot to take in, but there was something so alive and exciting happening there. New doors were unlocking for me.

I watched with wonder as many of my fellow students devoted themselves to a single approach. In the same way that teachers of traditional medicine are passionate that their protocols be followed to the letter, so are practitioners of other medical disciplines. Many homeopathic physicians (a medical science based on the principle of like curing like), naturopaths (a branch of medicine focusing on natural remedies to treat illness), and doctors of Chinese medicine (a holistic system based on living harmoniously with nature and continuously striving for balance, with the emphasis on prevention) and Ayurvedic medicine (a system of healing that originated in ancient India) also believe that their way is the only solution.

Our teachers were passionate and charismatic, and many of them had had personal success in their own disciplines. We looked to them for guidance and at times found it difficult to remain on neutral ground. The mission of the school was to teach an integrative approach to promoting wellness, and many of the students became fanatical about their course of study. Some of the classes also began to resemble personal therapy sessions, as it was the first time many of us felt heard and understood. It was difficult at times not to get drawn into other people's dramas, especially since all of us were searching for something.

I chose to remain on the periphery, observing and learning before deciding on my course of study. Eventually, I found what I was looking for and chose to be certified in multidimensional healing. This was what I believed in and desperately needed. One approach would not do it for me.

School thrilled me. The homework assignments stretched my mind and challenged me. Although some of the courses, such as anatomy and physiology, were extremely challenging, I couldn't wait to get to school and attend classes. I was sucking the information into me like a sponge and was beginning to understand my body and thought processes in a different way. I was curious to learn whatever I could about the connection between the body and the mind and about how one has the potential to influence the other. There had been a lot of sadness and frustration held inside my belly for such a long time that it started to be of little surprise to me that I had developed colon cancer. The point of my learning was not to inflict self-blame but to become aware of and alter patterns of behavior that were no longer benefiting me.

My daughters made fun of my new role as student. They could not imagine why I would choose to go back to school when they could hardly wait to be finished with it. We spent many hours studying and doing homework assignments together at the kitchen table. The three years were passing quickly. Jacqueline had already graduated from high school. She wore a beautiful white dress when she received her diploma, and all I could see were her eyes on me. My heart was full and my soul felt satiated. "One down, and two to go," I thought.

Very few students at the time had their own private practice. I was one of the lucky ones, having already taught creative visualization for a few years. As I continued to learn, my clients were also eager to share in my adventures. I had the wonderful opportunity to watch in real time the results of what I had been learning. This helped me find my own pathway toward healing. And it helped me become the kind of teacher I had always wanted to be. I was there to give my clients the space they needed, where all judgment was suspended. I advised them to view health care providers as resources. As long as they were getting their needs met, great, but when things changed, it was time to move on. At first, my clients were shocked by my bluntness. I told them that all therapists were there simply to provide a service. "It's a bonus if you happen to like us, but if you're worried about hurting our feelings because you don't feel that we are supporting you adequately, forget it. Seek help elsewhere!"

I encouraged my clients to learn, to study, and to explore. They needed to open themselves up and use a discerning eye if they were going to consider systems of medicine they had

never been exposed to. They needed to become active partic-
ipants in their health care process. They had to find out what
was right for them so that they could pick up that brush and
create their own story.

I LOVED WHAT I was doing. Working with people constantly
reminded me to walk my talk. I had developed a better awareness of my physical body and had an arsenal of tools and
strategies to help me cope with whatever came my way. Yet I
began to feel unsettled. Something wasn't right. Work was
going well. I had started lecturing and speaking at various
organizations about visualization and the power of the mind.
My kids and Jon appeared to be thriving. But there was a restlessness growing within me that was making me feel very
uneasy. Having gotten more in touch with my body, I knew
that something was amiss. I felt out of alignment, and I needed
to figure out exactly how and what to do about it.

I was unhappy as a vegetarian. I never really felt satisfied
when I ate. I craved hot dogs, french fries, and potato chips. I
was afraid to make any major changes to my diet, because it had
been more than four years without cancer rearing its ugly little head again, and somehow I had convinced myself that eating
this way would save my life. (You know the old adage "Don't
rock the boat"? Well, the boat felt pretty rocky all on its own.)

I was also still unhappy with my relationship with Jon's
mom. It was fine to tell myself that it was her problem and
that I shouldn't allow her actions to affect me. I understood
all of this on an intellectual level but still felt some of the same
internal anguish in my gut that I knew had contributed to
my getting sick in the first place. I began to realize she wasn't
what was making me sick; it was my inability to deal with her

that was the problem. I had given her my power and lost my voice in the process. I still had an innocent side that could not understand why she found me so difficult to get along with. I loved my husband and my children. Everyone seemed to be healthy and happy. Why wasn't that enough? Even my getting cancer did not soften her resolve. After my surgery for cancer, ten days passed before she visited. She told me that she didn't believe in bothering people when they were in the hospital. She was kinder to strangers than she was to me! I guess being the mother of her grandchildren didn't count for much. The ironic thing is, with my training in palliative care, I was the one who brought her to the hospital nearly twenty years later and cared for her when she was dying. I eventually grew to respect this strong, dynamic woman who I realized simply wanted to be loved and have a place in our lives. It was only on her deathbed that she said "Who would have ever believed it would be you taking care of me at a time like this? If I have ever done anything to hurt you, I am so sorry. Please forgive me."

Doctors may have been able to cut out the cancer, but as my mom once asked me, "Can they cut out the heartache at the same time?" How I wish it could have been so easy. But I was a work in progress. I knew I did not have all the answers, but I was going to continue to do my best to find them. I had so much to be grateful for. I just needed to keep reminding myself of that. I remember my daughter Kassy telling me what she had learned from listening to a lecture given by the Dalai Lama. He said that the biggest challenge we have in our lives is simply learning to be happy. This seemed straightforward enough in theory, but adopting it into practice was challenging for me.

(8)

HERE WE
GO AGAIN

IT WAS THE last quarter of my graduating year from the NHC Institute, and I was busy with term papers and exams. My daughters were eighteen, sixteen, and thirteen. They laughed and made fun of me when I told them I thought I might like to continue studying after school ended. I couldn't help it. I just loved what I was learning. Every day, I discovered something new. And with each discovery, more doors and opportunities seemed to open up for me. The possibilities appeared endless.

Jacqueline was already attending university, and I could hardly believe that Kassy would soon be graduating from high school. I had dreamed of remaining alive long enough to see them all graduate, and my dreams were being realized. I felt so blessed.

It was time for my annual checkup with my gynecologist. Here I was, forty-one years old, having had a hysterectomy at thirty-five. All I had left in my reproductive area was one lonely little ovary. Still, it deserved regular checkups. Following an unusually long examination, my normally jovial doctor looked genuinely shaken. He asked me to follow him right to the hospital, because he suspected something was very wrong.

I lay on the table while he did an ultrasound. My doctor said my ovary was now four times larger than its normal size and it had to come out immediately. I explained to him that my husband was in Israel and would be back ten days later. I refused to call Jon, and my doctor and I agreed to postpone the surgery until the day after Jon's return. My doctor never said the word, but I knew he feared it was cancer. My gut told me it wasn't, but I knew it wasn't going to be an easy ten days. I remembered how agonizing the waiting game was the first time around and prayed there would not be a repeat performance. I tried my best to get through that period by meditating, visualizing, and praying.

I greeted Jon at the airport with open arms and a smiling face. He chatted about his trip, and I did my best to listen enthusiastically. When he asked me how I was, I told him I was being operated on the next day because the doctor suspected ovarian cancer. His world crashed. All the joy he had experienced on his trip was gone in an instant. He swallowed hard as his eyes welled up with tears. Imploringly, he asked why I hadn't asked him to come home from Israel. That was a good question. I didn't know what to say. When I was eighteen and nearly died of mononucleosis, I wouldn't allow his mother to disturb his European adventure to tell him that news. When I was awaiting the colon biopsy, I didn't ask him to return from Toronto. Here I was, once again, on my own, not wanting to disturb his good time. Was I a saint, a martyr, or a complete idiot? I wasn't sure which.

I hadn't said a word to anyone about what was happening, as I thought Jon should be the one to hear the news first. It was difficult. I sought counsel from a homeopathic physician, who did her best to calm me so that I could function while I waited for him to return. When things are scary for me, or when I am dealing with a crisis, I put on a hat that reads "Functional Human Being." It is almost as though I have taken a giant zipper and zipped myself from top to bottom, preventing whatever precious energy I have within from leaking out. It's a survival instinct. I seem to be able to suspend emotion and simply go into action. I can't let myself feel for very long during these times, because I know that if I do, I will not be able to put one foot ahead of the other. It is only when a crisis passes that I give myself the space I need to breathe and process the events. I sometimes feel like the animal in the wild, moving instinctively toward survival and away from any sign of danger. My "zipping up" ensures that I keep my essence safe and protected. Only those closest to me suspect that something is up.

Although my gynecologist thought I was in trouble, something inside me knew I did not have ovarian cancer. I just couldn't shake the feeling, however, that something was amiss. After Jon spoke to the girls, he told me they thought not only that I was sick again but that this time I was dying. They had sensed a strong shift in my personality. They felt that I had become distant and withdrawn. To this day, they hate it when I retreat (though my eldest, Jacqueline, seems to have mirrored this behavior). They call me the ice queen. I refuse to emote during these times and appear to function robotically. The girls tell me that they can literally feel me withdraw my emotion and energy from them. It feels as though I have cut them off, and they don't like it. I do it to give myself space in which I can think without anyone influencing me. It is a way of keeping myself together in the face of adversity. Thank goodness my daughters had one another to talk to at the time, because none of them ever even approached me. I had always hoped that they would learn to count on each other, just in case I wasn't around. Although I hated the circumstances under which this happened, I was pleased that it did in fact occur. My daughters were angry and told me that I needed to stop trying to protect them. They had a right to know what was going on, they insisted. My behavior had filled them with anxiety, as they were anticipating the worst.

The surgery was a complete success, and we were all very relieved that the ovary was taken out before it had the chance to become cancerous. Its cellular makeup had already begun to change, and it might have been a problem in the future. I had to stay in the hospital for a few days, and the girls sat me down for a heart-to-heart. They explained that my trying to protect them by keeping my worries to myself was actually hurting them. If I was honest with them, then they could prepare themselves as best they could to deal with what they might have to face. If I hid what was going on, they had no way to get on with their lives. How could they feel free to make decisions about where to go to school or where to travel if they did not feel I was being honest with them? They needed to feel safe in order to thrive. I knew how important safety had always been to me and realized that for them safety meant full disclosure. It was time to come clean with both my husband and my kids. No more hiding, no more doing it all by myself. Although I still thought of them as my little girls, they were really young adults. It was time to start treating them as such.

A WEEK AFTER returning home from the hospital, I experienced my first bowel obstruction. I was so sick that I thought I was dying. I had been used to pain, but this was intense and beyond anything I could cope with. The day before, I had gone to see an acupuncturist whom I had known for years, to help me recover from the trauma of surgery. Worried that his treatment may have stimulated something that was now producing the pain, the poor guy came to the house to try to help me. He worked on me for hours without success. Not knowing at the time that it was a bowel obstruction, we figured something had gone wrong with the surgery. I lay in bed writhing like a wounded animal. Nothing I did could control the pain. Jon had to call an ambulance to get me to the Royal Victoria Hospital, where my gynecologist worked. I had always imagined that riding in an ambulance would be kind of fun. I can tell you that it was anything but. Every crack or bump in the road felt like a knife to my insides. The only comical moment was the look on the paramedic's face when I threw up all over him. Had I not been suffering so much, I might have laughed. But laughing at that moment was not an option. The pain was too severe.

I will never forget arriving at the emergency room. I was overcome with pain and lay there groaning loudly. A nurse aggressively yelled at me to be quiet and said I was being melodramatic and theatrical. Her words worked. She shocked me into silence. It was as if she had stuffed a cork into my mouth. The only evidence of my deep suffering came from an extremely elevated blood pressure, a contorted body, and tears pouring down my face. Surely, the nurse must have been pleased that I had stopped making so much noise so that her other patients were not disturbed! Jonathan and I were both so surprised by her actions that neither of us found our voice. We remained powerless.

A nasogastric tube was inserted, a chest X-ray was taken to ensure the tube was in the right place, and I was given morphine to make me feel more comfortable. The problem with a bowel obstruction is that nothing can be kept down. The naso-gastric tube suctions out any stomach contents, which could otherwise make me feel even more nauseous. Finally, I felt relief.

Just as I was about to fall asleep, the ER doctor in charge of my case marched into my little cubicle. He announced, "You have more serious things to worry about than a bowel obstruction. The chest X-ray shows you have lung cancer."

What? What did he say? What was wrong with this man? How could he just come in here and tell me that? I was not just angry; I was furious. How dare he make such a declaration without taking a biopsy? He explained that because of his many years of experience, he believed conclusively that I had lung cancer. He suggested I make arrangements with the oncologist who was treating me at Jewish General Hospital. What oncologist? It had been almost five years since my other cancer, and Alex Zukiwski had returned to Texas. What had happened to my ninety-five percent chance of disease-free living? I was stunned by the doctor's words.

I shrieked at the doctor to get out of my room and never come back. Moreover, I continued, as soon as I recovered from the bowel obstruction, I was going to leave his stupid hospital and never come back. I must have looked quite a sight. I was hooked up to an IV, there was a tube sticking out of my nose, and I was screaming like a bloody lunatic at a doctor who ultimately turned out to be right. But I just couldn't help myself. I was so upset. Jon was mute. Not a word came out of his mouth. He had turned ashen and was barely able to breathe, let alone speak. I had never seen him like this. He was para-lyzed with fear.

When I was diagnosed with cancer the first time, Jon asked the doctor what he could do to help me. He was told that if he really wanted to help, then he should do something to raise money for research. It would be through research that a cure would one day be found. So he started a race through the streets of Montreal called the Défi Canderel (the Canderel Corporate Challenge). One man alone could only do so much, but for the coordinator of a large-scale fundraising event, the sky was the limit. The first run took place in May 1990, after I was diagnosed with colon cancer, and as of today, the run has raised more than eight million dollars purely for research.

Jonathan may not have been able to fix me back then, but he put his heart and soul into creating something that might help eradicate this terrible illness. Now here we were once again. This time, he felt lost. He looked like a broken man. I tried to help. I tried to convince Jon not to believe the doctor. Wasn't it possible that whatever the doctor had seen on the X-ray was a fungus, or even tuberculosis? How the hell could he be so sure it was cancer? How could he tell me that without proof? Isn't that what medicine is all about: proof? Denial, I realized, even for a moment, can be a beautiful thing.

How I managed the nine long days in the hospital is beyond me. I remained isolated in a private room. I was beyond morose. I only left my room and walked the halls for a few minutes several times a day. There was nothing anyone could do for me. If the bowel obstruction did not reverse itself, I was told, I would require surgery.

Those days left me plenty of time to think. Very few doctors dared enter my room. The "Sweet Sucky Susie" of my previous lifetime became the "Angry Susan" who scared everyone. I lay in bed wondering if this really was going to be the end of my life. The words of that palm reader came back to haunt me. Could they be true? Was her prophecy unfolding before my eyes?

I had started volunteering in the palliative care unit at twenty-eight years old. Now, at forty-one, did I need assistance with the very thing I had helped others deal with? Was I going to die? I had never seriously thought I was going to die after the first surgery. I knew my life would be forever changed, but somehow, perhaps naively, I believed I would make it. This time, I wasn't so sure. I knew from my experience working at Hope & Cope that the odds of recovering from metastatic illness were not good. Cancer once was one thing, but twice was one step closer to the grave. Never in my wildest imagination could I have suspected lung cancer. Is that what my restlessness was all about? Did my body know long before my brain? I thought I had been doing so many wonderful things to help myself. Had it not been enough? Were health and well-being simply out of reach for me? I felt sad, disheartened, and alone. I was not sure what I was going to do. Was I ready to give up and let go?

I discovered later that when colon cancer spreads, ninety percent of the time it spreads to the liver. Only ten percent of the time does it go to the lungs. I wondered which was better. I remembered seeing the movie *The Doctor*, starring William Hurt, only a few months earlier, with my mom. The main character was depicted as a cold and detached physician. It was only later, once he developed throat cancer, that he softened, opened up, and allowed himself to be touched by his patients. His story moved me. I wondered at the time how personal traumas change our behaviors. I coughed throughout the entire movie, and with each cough, my mother cringed. "You have been coughing for over a month," she said. "Have that looked after." I said that I would but didn't bother, because I seemed to have that same allergic tickle in my throat every spring.

THE BOWEL OBSTRUCTION reversed itself after nine days. I was saved from abdominal surgery, but I wondered if I was being prepared for something much worse. I once heard someone say that as long as we are alive, pain is inevitable, but suffering is optional. At that moment, there appeared to be no options for me. My soul felt wounded, and my very essence was shaken to the core. As much as I hoped it wouldn't be true, somehow I knew it was: I had lung cancer.

I returned to the Jewish General Hospital and began testing in earnest once again. A biopsy had to be taken using something called fluoroscopic imaging. Dr. Max Palayew, chief of radiology at the time, performed the procedure. It was like watching a movie of my insides in real time. I could see how my rib cage moved with every breath. Then I saw it. It looked like a little white circle. The doctor asked me to hold my breath for as long as I could when he saw the tumor. He then inserted a needle and took a tissue sample. I was required to rest for hours afterwards to ensure that my lung did not collapse. Internal organs do not like being invaded. After the procedure was complete, the sadness in Max's eyes, as well as the gentle hug he gave me, confirmed what we'd suspected. I just lay there, quietly praying and asking God to hold my hand. Once again, I felt very small in that great big bed.

A couple days later, my eldest daughter, Jacqueline, came to the hospital with Jon and me to learn the official results. Cancer was confirmed. We met with a pulmonologist I had never seen before. She said that since adenocarcinoma of the colon looked so similar to adenocarcinoma of the lung, they could never be absolutely sure whether the cancer had spread from the colon or if it was a new one altogether. They were going to treat it as though it had spread. The doctor then proclaimed that if we did nothing, I would be dead within a year. She said that if we operated to remove the affected part of the lung, I would have a twenty-five-percent chance of living for five years.

The news was horrible to hear on my own, but having my daughter there cracked my soul. My insides melted in despair. It's a mother's role to protect her child, and here I was, being supported by her. She was calm and very quiet. I guess her mind was busy trying to figure out what she could do to help me. Only later did I find out that this was the moment when she chose to stay home rather than move out for her second year of college. She needed to make sure that I was all right. She selflessly put her own needs on the back burner.

Jon burst into tears. He has always been a sensitive person but manages to put on a brave face for the world. Here, sitting between Jacqueline and me, he could not even attempt to keep it together any longer. But I did not react. I simply listened to him weep as I discussed the options and statistics as if I were talking about a stranger's odds. Going numb was good for me. There was no way I was going to let myself feel. Just breathing felt like an aerobic exercise. It was difficult to think. Jacqueline was the one who comforted and hugged Jon. The thought of having anyone touch me at that moment disgusted me. Here it was again, an uninvited invader. How dare it take up residence in my lung? I had only smoked a few cigarettes, and that was in college. I felt repulsive and dirty inside. I realized how hard it must be to live with something that cannot be removed. No wonder we beg for surgery, even if it gives us only the smallest hope of survival.

Although my anger may have been misplaced, I decided that I hated this doctor too and would never see her again. How could she have been so cold and callous in the way she delivered the news? What was wrong with doctors, anyway? Where was their humanity? Hearing the words "I'm so sorry" or a gentle touch on my shoulder would have gone a long way. In hindsight, I probably would have hated anyone who delivered that news. Maybe the anger was my way of blaming someone for my situation. To help me get through this, I knew that I needed a doctor I could relate to. I'd had that experience with my surgeon and oncologist. I wanted someone who would partner with me in my journey and who was not afraid to get close. I was desperate for help and guidance. Handling the news was difficult enough, but I really did not want to feel that I had to handle my medical team as well. It was too much.

If I was going to go ahead with the surgery, then I had to put my anger and frustration aside. I needed to focus on the twenty-five percent of people who survive the five years. One in four seemed to be able to make it. What did they do? Whom did they seek help from? I was determined to put my efforts into figuring it out.

More tests needed to be done to determine whether the cancer had spread from one lung to the other. I met with a thoracic surgeon. He was kind but basically told me that if the cancer had spread to the other lung, surgery would not be an option. A mediastinoscopy (a diagnostic test to remove the lymph nodes from the sternum, the bone between the lungs) was scheduled for the following week. Dr. Nathan Sheiner suggested that I go to New York for the test. Memorial Sloan–Kettering Cancer Center offered a less invasive surgical option than the one used in Montreal. Dr. Sheiner figured that should I be eligible for surgery to remove the cancer, not dealing with two broken clavicles would make the recovery easier—in New York, the procedure was done through a small incision in the neck.

In the meantime, I was told to "relax and try to take it easy." What a joke! How could anyone take it easy at a time like this? What did taking it easy even mean?

I had been sliced and diced so many times, it was hard to imagine that I was going to go through it again. I joked with my husband, saying that if I ever had an affair it would have to be with a doctor, because only he could appreciate what a true medical marvel this body of mine was. I thought that was hysterical and could not stop laughing. Under the circumstances, Jon once again did not seem to share my sense of humor.

Chances were good that I would get to see Katherine graduate from high school, but what about Alexandra? She was only thirteen and had already seen me go through so much. I felt guilty. She had truly been shortchanged. When Jon asked her how she felt about the news that I had lung cancer, she flippantly replied, "How should I feel? Mom has been in and out of the hospital ever since I was born. She's always okay, and she'll get through this as well."

"Well, at least she isn't morose," I thought. I found out years later that Ali had asked her entire class to tape their fingers crossed together for good luck on the day of my lung surgery. She enjoyed the complete support of her teacher and classmates. They worked together, as a team, sending positive energy my way in the hope that I would make it. Only when she received the news that the surgery was a success did they un-tape their fingers. What an incredible support system Ali had by her side.

Katherine was a different story. She melted into a puddle. There was a part of her that I knew was too attached to me. As she would confide in me fifteen years later, she was thinking that if I died, she would die as well. For her own well-being, I knew that she needed to separate from me. Before this diagnosis, she had planned to go to France for a year of junior college. Keeping her home would have been a bad idea for both of us. She needed her freedom, and I needed time to heal without feeling guilty that I was keeping her from this incredible opportunity. She cried, not wanting to go, but I made her a solemn vow that I would call her back if things turned for the worse. I reassured my daughters that I would never hide anything from them again, and that if I ever needed them, I would let them know without hesitation.

I HAVE ONLY an obscure memory of what happened in the time between the tests and surgery. I do have some vague recollections of walking down the streets of New York with Jon and of him buying me a backless summer dress. I never wore that dress, as I was too shy to have the whole world see the scars on my back.

My niece Caroline visited me, as she was a medical student in New York at that time. She was there when a woman came into my room asking me whether I wanted to pray. I needed prayer like a thirsty flower in need of water. As we held hands together, I felt a sense of profound peace blanket me. I remember being impressed by Memorial Sloan-Kettering Cancer Center. It felt more like a hotel than a hospital.

Many other memories have been lost. I know that my unconscious mind must have been trying to protect me by covering up or hiding what was too painful to bear. What I do remember, however, is that when I awoke from the surgery, I envisioned a beautiful little flower in my driveway that breaks though a crack in the asphalt each and every spring. It chose life and with all the determination it could muster broke through what most would consider impossible circumstances. I clung to that image as I drifted off to sleep once again. I felt a smile crease my face. Maybe I would be like that little flower.

I returned to Montreal and awaited the test results. I never allowed myself to go to that place of wondering what I would do if they told me the cancer had spread. I figured that if I had to deal with that, I would have plenty of time when I got the news. In the meantime, I had enough to think about.

A few days later, I learned that the cancer hadn't spread to the other lung and that I would be able to proceed with the surgery. The doctors felt that this was great news and were encouraged. I was slightly cynical, since I'd been given a ninety-five percent chance of disease-free living the first time, and clearly the doctors had been wrong. I knew that there was no option for me other than surgery.

Although I hated the idea of being cut into again, I figured that this would be my best chance of getting to see my kids grow up, even if it was only for a short time. I was going to put into practice all that I had learned during the last five years. I was determined to become my own case study.

(9)

TO HELL
AND BACK

SURGERY WAS BOOKED for the following week: June 14, 1994.
One thing I needed to do first was go back to school and say
good-bye to my classmates. School was almost over, but I was
not going to be at my own graduation. I had previously missed
my high school graduation because I thought it was unimportant (I think the truth was that I did not have a boyfriend and
did not want to go to the party alone). I missed my university
graduation because I was too shy to show up seven months
pregnant, and now here I was, missing this one as well. It's
funny how patterns keep repeating themselves.

There were hugs. There were tears. All my teachers surrounded me in a prayer vigil. A fellow student shocked me
when she asked, "What do you think you did wrong to get cancer a second time?" I had already agonized over this question,
wondering if it would have made a difference if I had gotten
to that cough months earlier, and had decided that self-blame
was not helpful. Moving forward required a different approach.
I replied, "That's the wrong question. What you needed to ask

was what did you do right to keep it at bay for so long, and what more do you need to do to let it go once and for all?"

Wow! Where did these words come from? I rocked!

I guess I was preparing myself for the task ahead, a task that was going to be more difficult than anything I had ever faced before. This time, however, I was armed. God was by my side, along with a supportive family, good friends, a great medical team, and an arsenal of tools and strategies from healing modalities from around the world. I was as prepared as I was ever going to be. It was time to just get on with it.

The day of surgery is etched in my memory forever. This was going to be the day when they went inside my body to see what they could see. The results of this operation would probably determine whether I would live or die. There are no words to describe how I was feeling that early morning. As I was being wheeled to the operating room, I realized how different this cancer surgery felt from the first one. Back then, I was a scared little girl. This time, I wasn't scared; I was terror-stricken. The surgeon was going to crack open my chest. Practitioners of Chinese medicine believe that the chest is the place where the spirit resides. My spirit was now the only thing keeping me going. I hoped the surgeon wouldn't damage it. I remember praying, "Please God, hold me close, and even if I die, let me know that I am not alone."

My surgeon, Dr. Sheiner, informed me that he really did not know how long the operation would last. It would only be once he opened me up that he would be able to determine exactly what needed to be done. All I can remember him saying is that it would take longer to remove a part of a lung than an entire one. As I had done each and every time before surgery, I made the anesthesiologist promise that I would not wake up during the operation. I saw a movie once about someone waking up mid-surgery, and it traumatized me permanently. Now it was time to let go and allow what was to be to be.

I have no memory of interacting with anyone prior to the operation. To this day, I am still surprised when family and friends tell me they were there, sitting outside the operating room, supporting one another. I'm glad they had each other, because as painful as it was for me, I think it was even more difficult for them. They couldn't fix it, they couldn't make it better, and if there was any possibility I was going to die, they needed one another to lean on. That's what was going through my mind as I drifted off to sleep.

WHEN I AWOKE, I was very uncomfortable. I was in a lot of pain and had tubes coming out of me from everywhere. The respirator was the worst, and my reaction demanded that it be removed ASAP. I started hyperventilating and squirming; it made me feel like a caged animal. The nurses gave me something to stop the panic, and when I awoke again, the respirator was gone. "Imagine," I thought, "a machine was breathing for me." It was a difficult concept for me to comprehend. It made me feel subhuman.

The first thing I wanted to know was whether the surgery had been long or short. When Dr. Sheiner told me it had been short, I knew he had removed my entire right lung. He had found three tumors, not just one. "Good," I thought. "It's all gone. Good riddance." I decided then and there that I was letting go of any of the last remnants of cancer that may have been hiding in my body.

People came in and out of my room as I drifted between consciousness and unconsciousness, between wakefulness and sleep. My good friend Allen sent his best friend, Rubin Becker, who was a doctor at the hospital, in to check on me. (I had no idea then that he would end up being my doctor and dear friend some ten years later.) I remember smiling faces, bright lights, and noise, but not much more. Time was of no consequence to me then. I simply needed to get through each day. Breathing was difficult (and a few broken ribs resulting from the operation didn't help either), and everything hurt. I wondered how many body parts can be removed before a person dies. Would I really be able to function or quasi-function in spite of what had happened to me? Would I still look the same? What would keep my rib cage up? Could it just free float? What would happen to that empty space? Does it ever fill in? I'm not sure I ever voiced these thoughts; I just allowed them to float through my mind. "Time will reveal all the answers," I thought. I just had to wait and see.

Eventually, I must have left the intensive care unit, because I woke up in a regular hospital room. The first time I was operated on for cancer, I had received a ridiculous number of flowers, cards, and gifts. I'd had to ask the nurses to take the flowers out of my room, as the smell was overwhelming and my room began to look like a florist shop. This time was different. I received nothing. The contrast was glaring. I felt like a leper. Were people so scared that they didn't know what to do? Did they think I would die before I had a chance to enjoy any gifts? It was hard to believe that, with everything I was going through, this was what was on my mind. Perhaps the mundane was what I needed to take me away from the seriousness of my situation.

The hospital stay remains pretty blurry. What stand out most are the exquisite pain and the difficulty I had breathing. It wasn't supposed to be like this. The doctors said I had enough breathing capacity to make an easy transition from two lungs to one. I had done breathing exercises as part of stress management for years. I was an athlete, for heaven's sake, and now I could no longer take for granted the simple act of breathing, which was my birthright. I felt helpless. My breaths were shallow. I felt a hundred years old.

If we can base our present and future on past experiences, I assumed I would get over this and recover quickly. But I was dead wrong. I felt as though I had been run over by a truck, and no one had prepared me for that. I felt as though I had little control over my body, and I was beyond scared. I had no energy and was completely exhausted all the time. This was a far cry from the woman who thought that a five-mile walk was a good beginning. No one thinks about their body parts until something is wrong with them. How often do you think about your big toe unless you stub it? My thoughts were occupied entirely by my poor little lung and the trauma it must be feeling sitting all alone in my half-empty chest cavity.

AFTER A FEW weeks in the hospital, it was time to go home, but I did not want to. I did not feel ready. I was weak and fragile, a far cry from how I felt when I left the hospital after my colon surgery. I was afraid of my own body. I couldn't trust that it would function. We do, after all, have internal organs for a reason. I wasn't allowed to be alone for months. I suppose the doctors were concerned that I was not physically capable of being on my own. This is not particularly good for someone who needs a lot of personal space. I had to sleep on my left side so that my heart wouldn't move over too much (after all, there was nothing to stop it). I was given a lot of instructions to take home with me. There seemed to be way too many rules. I never questioned any of them; I simply complied.

Unlike the ride home after the first cancer, when I had been happy and excited to see everyone, this ride home was excruciating. I was tired from simply getting dressed, from being wheeled to the car. I wanted to cry, but that required energy, of which I had none. So I sat there like a lump, physically present and aware of every bump and crack in the road. Somehow, I made it home. I had to sit down five times before I reached the top of the staircase to my bedroom. Five times! Normally, I would easily run up the stairs, never even pausing for a moment. Now, after sitting down five times to catch whatever breath I had, I felt as though I had run a marathon. Coming home was no picnic. Sleeping was miserable, moving around was miserable, and life in general was miserable.

Kassy's high school graduation was a few days after I got home from the hospital. I knew I had to be there. No matter how terrible I felt, I had made a promise to her. I still remember the dress I wore: feminine and frilly. It had little flowers and soft pastel colors. When I saw myself in the mirror, I realized how awful I looked. The dress hung on me like a loose sack. I was slim to begin with, and losing fifteen pounds made me look like a plucked chicken. I have a very long neck, but now as the skin hung off it, I thought it looked as though it belonged more to a rooster than a woman. I laughed out loud when I thought what a picnic a plastic surgeon could have with me now. I was pale and exhausted, with huge bags under my eyes. Somehow, though, I managed to pull it off. It is amazing what a little bit of makeup can do. Jon had gotten permission from the school for us to come in through the side door of the gymnasium. He could park his car there so that I would not have to walk very far.

I will never forget what happened when he opened the door of the gymnasium. The ceremony was already in progress (thank goodness they did it alphabetically and "Wener" was almost last to be called). For a person who never loved the spotlight, it was disconcerting when all eyes turned toward me. Kassy's entire class stood up when they saw me, and I received a standing ovation. I did not know where to throw myself; I felt so exposed. I was overwhelmed and overcome with emotion. The gymnasium was completely full, and I was so grateful that someone quickly got up from his seat and gave it to me. I blissfully collapsed into it. I had made it! I'd promised Kassy I would, and I was able to keep that promise.

Tears fill my eyes as I write these words. I vividly recall the pride and the joy I felt being able to witness that event. No matter what had occurred, what was important to me was the fact that I did not break my promise. Where I found the energy to make it there is beyond me. I can only remember the fact that I was there. But, I wondered, would I be able to make it to Ali's high school graduation? It was three years away.

Kassy wanted to have a few friends come over to the house for a celebratory dinner after the ceremony. I waited in the car while Jon went to pick up food for dinner. I do not ever remember feeling so exhausted. I was tired to the bone. I was soaked with sweat and could barely breathe. There was absolutely nothing left in me. I was empty. Jon had to carry me up the stairs and help me out of my clothes. At that moment, I understood, on a deep personal level, why some people choose death. Living is at times just too difficult. I took some pills and cried myself to sleep. I may have missed the party, but I had made it to the main event.

My dad came over the next day. Not being allowed to remain alone was both a blessing and a nightmare. I have always been a private person (with the exception of my vegetarian stint). To this day, I cannot stand someone hovering over me or wanting to know my every move. Spending time with my dad was different. Never did I feel invaded by his presence. He knew how to simply be with me. He was the one my doctor found sitting outside my hospital room like a guard when I had my spine fused. He would not let anyone come in and disturb me. He was the one I could ask to help me bend my leg after a partial knee reconstruction. It didn't matter that I shrieked with pain; together we got that knee working. And now he was the one I so badly needed to curl up into to find my safe, sane place. I found myself gently weeping in his arms, telling him that I really didn't know if I had what it took to get through this. I told him that I wasn't sure I wanted to live. To wake up and feel this way every day was not living, to me. I knew that if I chose life, my battle was just beginning. At that moment, both life and death had an equal pull on me. It could have gone either way.

My dad held me and rocked me in his arms as if I were a small child. I felt wet from his tears. He told me that no matter what I chose, he would be there to support me. What a gift he gave me—the gift of unconditional love. Although I knew that he wanted me to live more than anything, he never did voice that desire. I was being heard, and it felt so good. I wasn't hushed up for thinking the unthinkable. He didn't offer suggestions. He simply allowed me to find my way, letting me know that I was not alone. I felt blessed and nurtured by his presence, cocooned and protected in his arms.

———

· *death* ·

IT IS VERY hard to discuss the subject of death with most people. Everyone wants you to live so desperately that they will accept whatever part of you is left, even if it is only a shell, as long as you don't leave them. But talking about dying doesn't necessarily mean you are going to die in the near future. In the West, death is not part of our regular education. It is hushed up and put on the back burner until we have no option but to face it. If I didn't have my sister, who is a trained therapist, and my dad to talk to, I think my journey into the possibility of death would have been much more difficult.

When I started working in palliative care, I wasn't afraid to walk into the room of a dying patient. There was something incredibly special about those people. The sheer honesty and purity of who they were deep down oozed out of their every pore. Sometimes, when I look in the mirror and put on makeup, I think that I'm covering up the "real" me. I have the ability to hide fatigue or a sallow complexion. Dying people have been stripped of all their window dressings. All you can see are their souls. I feel honored, not fearful, to be in their presence. They remind me to be real!

Many people ask me if I am drained or depressed working with people who face life-threatening illness. The truth is I am not. I am, however, often sad when they die. I miss their physical presence when they're gone. I felt that way when my dad died many years later. I crawled into bed with him after he died, etching the smell of him in my memory banks forever. Although I miss them, I am always grateful when their suffering is over. I feel blessed that they have trusted me enough to really get to know them. If I was able to offer them a moment of comfort, or an ear to listen to their concerns, I feel that I have done a good job.

I wonder if the sadness of loss might be a reason some doctors have difficulty getting close to their patients. If a cure is not in the cards, then they must feel like a failure when their patients are dying. But a cure is not the only thing we need from our doctors. A gentle touch or a warm embrace is sometimes all we require to help us feel connected and to ease the loneliness of our journey. All doctors can do, after all, is offer the best of their trade to their patients. It is up to the patients' bodies to determine the outcome. Once doctors understand this concept, I imagine the huge burdens they carry on their shoulders might be lightened, and perhaps their humanity could have more of an opportunity to shine. The truth is that what we gain from giving of ourselves is far greater than any potential loss!

(10)

NOW WHAT?

NOT LONG AFTER the surgery, I went to the country with my husband. He was eager to show me the completed interior renovations of our cottage, which we had agreed to do the previous fall, before I got sick. He was bursting with pride. He loved the country. It was his place to reconnect to his soul and let go of the worries of day-to-day life. But as I walked through the house, I told him that if I should die, he would have a really easy time sharing his home with another woman since nothing about it reflected me. I know that it was a horrible thing to say, and my words crushed him. But at the time, I didn't really care. I am a city girl, and I did not want to heal in the country, but because I was not allowed to be alone, I had no choice. Jon had thought that he would work from the country for the summer, enabling me to have a peaceful place to gain back my strength. He made sure that there was always someone with me if he had to return to the city for any reason. The only problem with his decision was that this was Jon's safe place, not mine. If I was mean, it was too bad. He would have to deal with his hurts and disappointments on his own. I was nobody else's therapist at that moment.

My doctors told me to take at least three months off work. I had nothing to do except think about me. I was in the depths of pure narcissism, and I relished it. Look at that—finally, I came first.

The kids were away at summer camp, and all I knew was that I was stuck in the country for the summer. How could I heal in a place I barely recognized? I knew I was depressed, and truthfully, I was rarely depressed. These were foreign feelings to me. I may be a happy and content person by nature, but what I needed now was to explore that dark and dreary place. I had always encouraged my clients to go there if they needed to, but then get out. I found myself stuck there, reveling in the muck like a pig playing in mud. There was a part of me that needed to really understand what misery and anguish felt like.

My days seemed endless. Jon was happy helping landscape our property. He was getting his needs met and was probably thrilled to be away from my gloomy presence. I was not exactly fun to be with. I watched him closely from my window. He is a big man, but he moved around easily and effortlessly. He loved the hard work. Chopping trees and digging trenches were therapy for him. He could go on for hours, sweating and loving every minute of it. I am long and lean, and I found myself exhausted just walking around the house. I both envied and resented his well-being. I had always taken good care of myself, whereas he simply ate and drank whatever he wanted. How could I be the one who got sick? For the first time in my life (and I hope the last), I truly felt that life wasn't fair. I felt like a lost lamb, weak and vulnerable, and oh so very sorry for myself. I needed to mope and bemoan my fate. Thank goodness I had my dog, Scruffy, for no matter how miserable I was, she thought I was perfect.

I stayed in this dark, bleak place for more than a month, until one day I couldn't take it anymore. We must have had twenty people working on the property daily. There was constant noise from morning until night. Privacy was difficult for me to find. One evening, I took my first post-surgery bath. It had been well over a month since I was able to bathe, and it felt like an eternity. The wait was finally over. I lit some candles and placed them all around the tub. I dimmed the lights, turned on some quiet music, and could hardly wait to get in. Bathing is one of my favorite things to do. Whenever I travel, I try to find a hotel with a bathtub. I must look like an actress in a television commercial advertising bubble bath. As soon as I slip into the tub, I can feel all my aches and pains begin to drain away from me. I become peaceful and calm. Even if I only have five minutes, it is well worth it.

Within moments of sinking into the tub, I felt myself, at last, becoming tranquil. Much to my chagrin, not five minutes later, a bright light shone through the bathroom window directly over my body. I let out a blood-curdling yell. Jon had organized for night lighting to be placed high in the trees to give the property a magical feeling. Of course, it could only be installed and tested at night. Outside my drapeless windows was a team of men setting up the lighting. I quickly crawled out of the bathtub and slithered along the floor to exit the bathroom. I felt that there was no hope for me. I so desperately needed peace and quiet.

The next day was a Friday. I tried to have a quiet breakfast, but some machine was making so much noise that I could not contain myself any longer. There are times when anger is really good. In this case it was what I needed to push me into action. At about 11 a.m., I called Jon into the house and I became completely hysterical. Perhaps he thought I was being irrational, but it didn't really matter. All I knew was that if I did not have everyone, including him, leave immediately, I was going to have a nervous breakdown. I told him that I didn't care if he had to pay the men their full day's wages, they just all needed to get out, and to get out now. I must have really scared him, as the look in my eyes made him realize that I was not kidding around. Like a little boy, he asked me where he should go. I told him that I didn't care, but he just had to leave. He made me promise to call him if I wasn't well. Knowing it was the only way to get rid of him, I agreed.

There it was: peace at last. I closed the gates around the property and, for the first time in a month, sat outside, quiet and alone. It was so beautiful. I had never noticed all the work Jon had done. He was creating an oasis for me. It was to be my own private sanctuary, a place to go when I needed to feel whole. I was so busy being angry and self-absorbed that I had missed the point of everything he was trying to do. All the trees, all the bushes, all the greenery were filling my poor little lung with oxygen and life force. I know in my soul that this was the moment when I chose to live. I proceeded to cry for two hours, pounding the ground and singing, "I am alive as the earth is alive. I have the power to create my freedom." Over and over again, I sang, until I had no more breath. And for the first time since the surgery, I fell into a beautiful, peaceful sleep right there on the grass.

SO I HAD decided I needed to live, but now what? It was roughly four and a half weeks post-surgery, and I was still quite fragile. I hated seeing myself this way. It was time to get down to business and climb out of my hole. I looked like a scrawny little girl. I needed healthy food, fresh air, and a good pair of running shoes. My first walk was only for a third of a mile. I huffed and puffed like an old woman but was very proud of myself. I was dealing with a bunch of broken ribs, so anything that rubbed against the incision hurt. I had to go braless for the first time in my life and felt like quite the rebel. Just the thought made me giggle.

That night, I wanted some semblance of normalcy, so I decided it was time to get intimate. It had been a long time, and sexless living was not for me. I was on a mission. I bathed, creamed my body, and with great determination tried to seduce my husband. Poor Jon was terrified. He didn't know where, or even how, to touch me. Everything hurt, but I pretended to whimper with delight instead of pain (I do not think he was fooled). The entire episode should have been a *Saturday Night Live* skit, because it really was quite contrived.

Then I heard the sound. It was a sound I will never forget. It sounded like a glug, glug, glug, swishing back and forth. You know the sound you might sometimes hear when you have had too much to drink and your belly feels like it's jiggling full of water? I was stunned. I first thought the sound was coming from outside my bedroom window. I was mortified when I realized it was emanating from inside my now half-empty chest cavity, and I burst into tears. I was filled with some sort of liquid. This was a sound I had never heard before. It was confirmed. I was a freak, some sideshow in a circus! Why didn't anyone warn me? Was this subject taboo? Did my doctors think that sex was no longer a possibility for me, just because I had one lung? Could they not have prepared me in some way? Surely, I was not the first person to experience this. I already had to adapt to so many changes, and I had no idea what I was going to do about this. I felt embarrassed and humiliated. All I had wanted was to feel normal. This episode confirmed for me that everything I had considered at one time to be normal would never be so again. It was an extremely painful realization.

Many questions flooded my mind, and I required answers. I needed to know if I was going to sound like a babbling brook for the rest of my life. I knew that I had to sleep on my left side for three months so that my heart wouldn't move over too much, but then what? How were my ribs going to stay up without my lung? What would fill that space? Would the liquid remain there forever? Bodies were not built to exist without internal organs. My doctors did not have many answers for me. I was basically told to be patient, that all the answers would be revealed in time (which I suppose meant they did not have a clue), and that this was all part of the healing process. Their responses disappointed me, and I came to realize that I would have to find out the answers on my own.

I might have appeared normal to the outside world, but I knew there was nothing normal about my insides. I could not escape myself. It didn't matter what Jon did or said. He could not relieve my misery. The only time I found true solace was with God and my dog, Scruffy. To them, I was still whole, no matter what was taken away from me. To them, I was perfect. As far as sex went, for now it was definitely out. I was not ready for any part of it. It would be a few months before I would venture to try it again. As the old adage goes: time really does heal all. I learned that I had an amazing ability to adapt to new situations, and in time, I learned to thrive once again.

Once I make up my mind to do something, I rarely look back. Being disciplined by nature, I knew that I would have to work really hard to become physically active once again. I think the reason I loved dance so much was that movement was effortless for me. I never thought of it as exercise. I thought of it as freedom! Since I was no stranger to pain, and no one told me not to, I pushed my body until I could barely breathe, rested a bit, and then pushed it some more. Sometimes my heart was beating so rapidly, I thought it would literally jump out of my chest. I was not just Susan Wener, a woman recovering from lung cancer. I became Susan Wener, a living, breathing science experiment.

Day by day, I gathered my strength. I thought I was doing really well until I heard myself on a telephone answering machine. I sounded breathless after just a few words. My inhalations echoed loudly, and I whistled and wheezed as I spoke. Not great for someone who did a lot of public speaking. I wondered if those days were over. Was I going to be reminded of lung cancer every time I spoke? Would everyone I talked to immediately know that something was out of sorts? First it was my hair that I thought gave me some kind of anonymity. Now what would keep me from being continuously exposed? Was I going to have to redefine myself once again? How many more adjustments was I going to have to make? I was curious about how the doctors were able to determine that I would be fine following the removal of my right lung. Just because a person can live with only one lung doesn't mean everything will be fine.

About four months after the surgery, my empty rib cage collapsed. I could barely look at myself naked in the mirror, as one side of my chest was indented a full two inches. I looked lopsided but was grateful that I was able to hide it with my clothing. I was always shy about my body, but this was no longer about being shy. I felt deformed. My doctors told me that eventually things would return to normal. I wasn't waiting to see if they were right. I went to see a wonderful osteopath who told me that the rib cage was compressing my liver. I worked with her for over three years two to three times a week to eventually put it back in place. But according to the doctors, I was doing just fine because I was indeed breathing! They have no idea how each little bump in the road adds up, making recovery a trying ordeal.

Sometimes, in the quiet moments, I remembered the words of that palm reader who told me at the age of twenty-seven that I would have a life filled with illness and then die young. Those words no longer kept me up nights as they had so long ago, but somehow they never left my memory bank either. If an early death was to be my fate, then I was determined to live each moment fully while I was still here. I would not live a wasted life. I would not bemoan my fate. I needed to find the strength to go on, no matter what the outcome. Someone once said that healing begins when treatment ends. Physically, I was mending well; now it was time to place my attentions on healing mentally and emotionally.

THE SUMMER PASSED, and I was called into my new oncologist's office. After reviewing my case, the tumor board recommended chemotherapy. "Here we go again," I thought. I refused to follow the doctors' advice and determined that this time chemotherapy was not for me.

My doctors were frantic. I was only forty-one years old. They were scared that I would die. My first oncologist, who no longer worked in Montreal, called me from Texas to try to persuade me. My surgeon also called me. But my husband had my back and supported my decision. Try to imagine this scenario: Doctors begging me to take chemotherapy, meeting my husband behind my back, hoping to convince him to influence me. A husband barely hanging on, knowing that a second cancer was one step closer to the grave. And me refusing to listen to medical advice. Was I in denial? Did I have a few screws loose? Had I lost touch with reality completely? I don't think so. This time I did my homework. There was absolutely no statistical data available that indicated I would receive any benefit from chemotherapy once the lung had been removed. My decision to do chemotherapy after my colon surgery had not prevented me from getting cancer a second time. There was no way I was going to put my body through chemotherapy just because the doctors could offer me nothing else. I was steadfast in my beliefs. Nothing anyone said would make me change my mind. I decided that the lung was the last remnant of any existing cancer in my body. Although some of those around me thought I was in la-la land, I felt myself firmly planted on the ground. I had a strength and determination growing inside me that had never existed before. I kept thinking that I needed a different approach from the one the doctors were offering me. In Chinese medicine, health is determined by balancing all of the organs within the body, along with the mind and spirit. When all systems are in balance, it is difficult for illness to exist. I was looking to shift the imbalances that may have allowed the cancer to spring to life and take root in my body in the first place. I needed to get to the source. Something was missing from Western medicine. Why were my blood tests always perfect? Why couldn't the diagnostics used by traditional medicine warn me of irregularities long before three tumors were discovered in my lung? Here I was again, with so many questions. I wondered if they could ever be answered to my satisfaction.

I had decided to go rogue, and from the moment I made my decision, I never looked back. I was not afraid. If I was going to die, I was going to die my way. I was quite peaceful. I thought that I had come to terms with the idea of death long before. What I came to realize, now that its possibility loomed before me once again, was that the concept of death is like peeling an onion. With each layer comes a different understanding. I am not sure that I will ever truly understand them all until death becomes my personal experience, and perhaps not even then. What I am left with are moments of fear. I have learned to not be defined by them. I simply watch and notice as they change with each new experience.

When I was eighteen, I nearly died from mononucleosis. I was sick for more than six months. There is not much you can do to treat that disease, and rest is usually the only medicine. I developed secondary infections in my ears, nose, and throat. Eating became impossible. I am five-foot-five and generally weigh about 115 pounds. I was so sick that my weight plummeted below eighty pounds. Just before I was transported to the hospital, I had a strange out-of-body experience. I did not see God, or that notorious white light. But I did realize in that moment that my consciousness was on the ceiling, and I felt myself watching the entire scene from above. Nothing hurt me any longer, and I was fully aware of everything that was happening. I saw my small body lying in my parents' big bed. My mother was crying, but I felt fine. I was semiconscious and unable to tell her that I was all right. It was then and there that I decided that one day I would work with people who were seriously ill.

———

· *the space between* ·

WHEN WE ARE sick, we spend far too much time worrying about whether we will live or die. It would make so much more sense to think about how well we could live, or even how well we could die.

Death is inevitable. We cannot hide from it. We will never escape it. It is a part of the human condition. This doesn't mean, however, that we cannot enjoy our lives, even if death appears closer than we might like.

I find it very interesting that when we go to a cemetery and look at a tombstone, the date of birth and the date of death are what appear most prominently. Everything that exists for us, however, takes place in the space between the two. That's where our focus needs to be: in the space between.

(11)

UNCHARTED WATERS

THE DECISION NOT to do chemotherapy showed me how much I was changing. I used to tell my children that they would know they had grown up when they listened to what was said, assessed it, and then decided whether it fit into their view of the world. After serious consideration, irrespective of whether anyone agreed with their decisions, they needed to do what made sense to them. I was beginning to follow my own advice. The old Susan would have crumbled under the mounting pressure. She wouldn't have wanted to disappoint anyone. I finally realized that I did not need to please anyone other than myself. Although my choice might affect the lives of those around me, they would have to deal with that on their own. This was my life and, therefore, these would be my choices. I was prepared to deal with whatever consequences I had to face. I found myself grounded, propelled forward with a newfound confidence. Instead of wanting to move away from cancer, I began moving forward. I went from reading books about cancer to reading books about health and well-being. I no longer wanted to be defined as a cancer patient.

I noticed that my children seemed to follow my lead. If I was okay, they were, too. My eldest daughter said, "You do what you need to do, Mommy. If you die, I want you to know that you live inside me, and all the lessons you've taught me will carry me through my life. I will always hear your voice." That was a pretty incredible thing for a nineteen-year-old to say.

Although I was disappointed that I could not seem to find a whole person holistic approach to healing in any one place, I was generally satisfied with the medical care I had received. I was offered the best available at the time. I went for checkups every three months for the first two years after lung surgery. My reaction to these routine checkups was interesting to me. Although I was comfortable with my decision to forgo chemotherapy, I was terrified whenever the time came for my appointments. I would not sleep for a week beforehand and found myself to be jumpy and short-tempered. I almost felt as though the doctors were checking me out to see what was wrong. My husband used to tell me I was behaving as though I had my period. I wanted to shoot him when he said that (especially since I had not had my period since I was thirty-five), but I have to admit it was true. I was nervous and irritable. Somehow I needed to convince myself that I was going to the doctor to show him how fabulous I was. I figured he needed that, since so many of his patients were not doing well. It was hard work, but I made a conscious decision that I was going there for wellness testing. I was there to let them see how well I was progressing.

My challenge was to create a healthy internal environment that would not support cancer. I wanted to become so healthy that there would not be any room for it to grow again inside this body of mine. That was quite a tall order, but I had to get down to the cellular level in order to make the necessary changes. Although I will never know for sure if any or all of the things I tried had a role in my being alive more than twenty-four years after colon cancer, what is most important to me is that I believed in what I was doing. I felt responsible to, and for, myself. My attitude affected my conduct, and it encouraged me to continuously strive toward health and well-being. I know that some people (including a few of my doctors) thought I was out of my mind. Others were playing the wait-and-see game. They were waiting to see if cancer came back, and if it did, wondering whether I would return to a more traditional model of medical care.

I decided that I was not going to hold back. I was determined to try everything and anything I could, as long as it made sense to me. I am grateful to this day that my doctors didn't dump me. They were still prepared to monitor my progress, even though I may not have chosen to follow their advice.

I was faced with the difficult task of trying to figure out what would benefit me most. There were so many options out there, many of which were not accepted by the traditional medical community. I had to navigate these waters on my own, hoping that I would make decisions that were good for me. Today, there is much more information available about complementary and alternative medicine, and the idea of incorporating it into one's health care program, although not mainstream, is more easily accepted than it was back then.

————

· *CAM* ·

MOSBY'S MEDICAL DICTIONARY defines what is today called CAM (complementary and alternative medicine) as a large and diverse set of systems of diagnosis, treatment, and prevention based on philosophies and techniques other than those used in conventional Western medicine, often derived from traditions of medical practice used in other (non-Western) cultures. Such practices may be described as an alternative that exists as a body separate from and as a replacement for conventional Western medicine, or complementary, that is, used in addition to conventional Western practice. CAM is characterized by its focus on the whole person as a unique individual, on the energy of the body and its influence on health and disease, on the healing power of nature and the mobilization of the body's own resources to heal itself, and on the treatment of the underlying causes, rather than symptoms, of disease. Many of the techniques used are the subject of controversy and have not been validated by controlled studies.

——

It is difficult to evaluate exactly what it was that made me feel better. Sometimes just knowing that you are doing something, anything, may contribute to an enhanced sense of well-being. I had armed myself with many tools in the previous five years that helped me deal with the mental and emotional aspects of cancer. I was writing regularly, practicing meditation and visualization, eating well, and having regular appointments with a massage therapist, an osteopath, and a doctor of Chinese medicine. I became a voracious reader and spent hours in bookstores. My home started to resemble a bookstore itself, shelves stacked high with books about all aspects of health and well-being. I used to tell Jon that I was high maintenance—but not in the way you might imagine. I didn't constantly go the hairdresser or buy expensive clothes or jewelry. I did, however, spend most of the money I earned from my private practice on myself. It felt really good to take care of myself, and it was exciting to see how well I felt. School had opened my eyes to other systems of medicine (Chinese, homeopathic, naturopathic, Ayurvedic, and energetic) and helped me understand that illness has effects over and above the physical ones. I loved the idea that thought or touch or intention could influence health.

——

· *energetic medicine* ·

REIKI, AS DEFINED by the *The Free Dictionary* by Farlex, is "a form of therapy that uses simple hands-on, no-touch, and visualization techniques, with the goal of improving the flow of life energy in a person. Reiki (pronounced *ray-key*) means 'universal life energy' in Japanese, and Reiki practitioners are trained to detect and alleviate problems of energy flow on the physical, emotional, and spiritual level." Reiki touch therapy achieves similar effects to those of traditional massage therapy—stress and pain relief and reduction of the symptoms of a variety health conditions.

Therapeutic touch is defined by *Merriam-Webster's Medical Dictionary* as "a technique often included in alternative medicine in which the practitioner passes his or her hands over the body of the person being treated and that is held to induce relaxation, reduce pain, and promote healing."

Qigong is defined by *Webster's* as "an ancient Chinese healing art involving meditation, controlled breathing, and movement exercises designed to improve physical and mental well-being and prevent disease."

———

But which path was I to choose? I had already seen when I had colon cancer how many people were willing to offer advice. Everyone knew someone who had tried something. I went from naturopath to naturopath, from healer to healer, and from dietician to dietician, trying to find my way. There was little consensus among therapists, and I often left my sessions feeling even more confused than when I had walked in.

I will never forget one professed healer I saw. I had heard that he laid hands on you and was able to calm your anxiety quickly. I figured that this could only benefit me. He lived quite far away, and in order to make my appointment on time, I gave myself a full hour to get there. I arrived at his door about ten minutes early and, with a bit of hesitancy, rang his doorbell. When he answered, he looked me straight in the eye and said that it was "just as rude to be early as it is to be late." He told me to "go and sit down somewhere" while he finished his tea. That certainly set the tone for our session. I was mortified. He then told me that he determined his fee structure after he assessed the client visually. He decided that I must pay the maximum fee. He said all of this before he even said hello! I just sat there, speechless and absolutely terrified.

When I returned home, Jon asked me how it went. I could not even tell him a thing about the session. I don't think I heard a word the "healer" said to me. How I wish I'd had the courage to get up and leave. Today, I would have told him where to go and walked out the door. Then, I acted like a scared little rabbit. I realize now how much of my power I gave over to him that evening and how potentially damaging some people can be.

—————

· *a third ear* ·

WHEN WE ARE vulnerable and looking for answers, we find ourselves swimming in a sea of possibilities. Some may serve us well, and some may not. It is hard to listen and make good decisions during these times. It is important to have another pair of ears listening, because when we are nervous, we often do not hear everything that is being said. People who believe passionately in what they are doing can easily sway us one way or the other.

When you first meet with a healer, or someone who is introducing an option you know little about, it is very important to bring along someone who can offer objective counsel. If the practitioner refuses to allow the other person in the room, it is then time to leave. If you must visit a healer by yourself, record the conversation so that you can listen to what they say without trying to write down or remember everything.

I also advise my clients to go home, assess what has been said, and see whether the treatment makes sense to them. Should there be products to buy, never buy them on the spot. Go home and think carefully before making any hasty decisions. There will always be time to buy products later. Don't get carried away and end up without rent money because you were swayed by a charismatic therapist!

—————

It scares me to think how easily I could have harmed myself throughout my adventures. I have gotten caught up many times in the energy of a supposed expert. I was so hungry for anything that could potentially save me. I was vulnerable and willing to try it all. I put my faith in questionable practices, as well as in supplements that I had absolutely no business putting my trust in. There were times when my husband told me I could have opened my own pharmacy. Most of the products ended up dumped into my garbage can. I was not able to stomach the sheer quantities of vitamin and mineral supplements that were suggested.

I can't stress enough the importance of research. Today I refuse to listen to someone's advice without carefully reviewing it. Once upon a time, I would have blindly done anything if I felt there was some hope in it; now I know that one thing does not cure all, in spite of what the Internet may say! The body is complex. Our internal organs work as a team. Too much of any one thing can easily upset the entire system. I have learned that less is often more, and I take very few supplements on a regular basis. I try my best to eat well and vary my diet so that I get the nutrients I need from real food rather than from pills.

A lesson I learned after trying one distasteful treatment (drinking my own urine) was to never blindly agree to anything without doing careful due diligence. This is more challenging than it seems, and because a treatment works for one person does not mean it will work for you. We often do not make the best decisions when we are in a vulnerable state. I love the expression "Trust in God, but tie your camel to the post." In other words, carefully examine your options. Then, once you have determined the best course of action for yourself, believe in what you are doing. Having your belief system in alignment with your actions will only enhance your journey toward health and well-being.

————

· *supplements* ·

MANY OF US spend an awful lot of money trying whatever supplement is popular at the moment. This product will make us thin, while that one will keep us youthful. One pill will cure illness, while the next one will help us remember the reason why we are taking all the pills!

Unfortunately, most of the time all we are doing is producing some very expensive urine. We need to ensure that we do not create other health conditions because of excessive supplementation. The availability of so many supplements to the general public must terrify doctors. This might be one of the reasons they don't trust many alternative medical practitioners. Watching some patients abandon Western medical practices in order to dive into that poorly regulated "other world" must be worrisome.

Although it is true that some of what we try might be harmful, doctors need to understand the motivation behind what we are doing. A cancer diagnosis is daunting. Western medicine often makes us feel horrible Sometimes the treatments we take can be toxic and might even kill us before the cancer does. Being physically sick from chemotherapy was not exactly my idea of a good time. I was leading a somewhat surreal existence. I functioned to the best of my ability between treatments and slept or puked for the five days during them. Had my mind not aided me by disappearing and daydreaming, I'm not sure how I would have made it through.

Aside from the physical discomforts that may arise from treatment, doctors simply do not have the time to deal with all of the emotional aspects we may simultaneously be trying to sort out. Turning to those who do have the time and who can offer us guidance is a no-brainer. I wish I had the knowledge then that I have now about who to talk to or where to go for help. I desperately needed guidance. Today, I help my clients navigate that mysterious world of alternative medicine. We often hunt together to find options that will help make their journey easier. I also advise my clients to access whatever is offered in their hospitals and their community centers. No one needs to travel this journey alone.

———

WHILE DECIDING ON my action plan, I discovered that Quebec has a huge underground network in the field of alternative medicine. There are all kinds of practitioners and healers providing services that exist beneath the surface of what is considered "allowable." Everyone knows that we can cross the border into Mexico, as well as Central and South America, to obtain questionable (and sometimes very effective) treatments, but I soon realized that I didn't have to travel very far, as these treatments exist right here where I live.

I read an article from the *Boston Globe* one day about a teenage boy who decided to go "underground to Canada" for alternative cancer treatments. Chemotherapy made him feel so sick that he told his parents he would prefer to die than continue it. It was a newsworthy story, as the U.S. government tried unsuccessfully to intervene and force him to continue treatment. His parents supported him completely, and together they traveled to Quebec. One of the things he tried was a product called 714x, a mixture of camphor, nitrogen, and sea salts. After he used this product for an undisclosed period of time, his cancer was put into remission.

I decided that I wanted to try the same product. One of the first things I had to do as part of the protocol was have my blood tested. I had it done at a lab in Rock Forest, Quebec. Even though I was frightened, I went to the lab by myself and never even told my husband until it was over. I did not want anybody to influence my decision. I wondered what the lab technicians would see when they examined my blood and what they would suggest. The memory of the palm reader's dire prediction came back to haunt me once again. I did not want a repeat of that experience.

I never understood why the blood tests I had every three to six months were unable to pick up any irregularities or signs of illness. How was it possible to have cancer, not once but twice, and still have all indicators appear perfectly normal? Well, not this time. My blood seemed to tell a tale all its own. I had never had what is called a "live blood" analysis before, and I saw things that were completely foreign to me. The technicians performing the test (just a simple pinprick) told me that they could see that I had had cancer and explained in detail what they saw in my blood. They even gave me a videotape of what they had seen under the microscope. It was a really weird experience. I felt as though I was looking at something out of a science fiction movie. My blood did not look anything like I had seen in medical textbooks. It looked like it was filled with debris. My red blood cells appeared to be clumped together and "sticky," rather than free-flowing. As scared as I was about what the tests might show, I was also relieved that finally somebody could see that all was not well within me. Playing the wait-and-see-if-cancer-came-back game was not my style. I needed to be proactive, and I finally had something to work with.

When I relayed my experience to Stephen Carson, he thought I had gone off the deep end. He could not understand what the technicians who read the test were talking about. He told me that he was trying to keep an open mind but that I should be very wary about this protocol; he urged me not put all my hopes in one basket. If Stephen thought I was out to lunch, I didn't dare imagine what my oncologists might think. My intuition had rarely been wrong in the past, and I felt completely in alignment with what I was doing. It did not matter to me if the entire world thought I was nuts. It was my understanding that 714X was not meant to cure cancer. It was supposed to help clean and purify the blood. It made sense to me that if my blood was healthy, cancer would not have an environment to thrive in. The Princess Margaret Cancer Centre in Toronto had some ongoing 714X trials at that time, and I was able to get the product for free from a reputable medical doctor. I bought a bunch of needles at the pharmacy and injected myself in the groin with 714X every evening. The protocol was an injection every day for twenty-one days. You then needed to stop for three days and repeat the cycle until further tests showed the blood to be clean and free flowing, according to the specifications of Gaston Naessens, the inventor of 714X. I did this routine for nine months.

But I did not do this blindly. I did a lot of research on Gaston Naessens, long before I ever went to his laboratory. Upon researching him, I discovered that my own oncologist had been part of a group that evaluated 714X and found it ineffective (imagine what he might think if I told him that I was trying it). Naessens was accused of practicing medicine without a license (he was a biochemist, not a physician) and was even implicated in a few deaths. (I think some very ill patients abandoned Western medicine in favor of 714x as a last-ditch effort to save their lives, and died in the process. There is no evidence proving they wouldn't have died anyway.) Eventually, Naessens was acquitted on all counts, but McGill University and all its affiliated teaching hospitals in Montreal refused any attempts at a clinical trial with this product.

I now faced a huge dilemma. For my sanity, I needed to fully believe in the product, and I decided to keep what I was doing hidden rather than allow my doctor to dampen my enthusiasm. It was only sixteen years later, when I collaborated with my oncologist on an integrative health series, that I admitted to him what I had done. His thoughts on the matter had not shifted one iota. I tried to explain why I did what I did, but he was not interested and remained steadfast in his beliefs. Today, many people think that 714x has no benefit for cancer patients. I never looked at it as a cure. I looked at it as a way of cleaning my blood, and hence was not disappointed. Trying 714x was one thing. After my doctor's reaction, I certainly wasn't going to tell him about any of the other things I'd tried. It was interesting to note that although he thought this product was "garbage," there were no irregularities in my blood tests (other than what appeared to be a slight allergic reaction to something) during a time period spanning two to three years when I experimented with a variety of products. It was therefore easy for him not to suspect I was doing anything that might cause him concern. All these years later, I did not need my doctor to accept 714x as something that may have helped me; I was simply hoping that he would understand why I had not revealed my choices to him at the time.

———

· *support* ·

SUPPORT IS AN essential ingredient of optimal health. Support systems can include anyone we trust and can go to for help or advice. The support we get often determines how well we deal with life's challenges. We need to surround ourselves with those individuals who can help us alleviate our stress so that we can better face what lies ahead. Support groups often fill this role— those who face similar challenges can often be our best guides. It is so important to have our doctors' support and encouragement as well. They must understand that we will use whatever treatments, therapies, or strategies make sense to us so that we can live fullest and richest lives possible.

For some, this could mean hours in the garden, whereas for others, it could mean meditating in the Himalayan mountains. The more we feel we are doing to help ourselves, the better our quality of life. That does not mean that we go against medical advice just to make our point. It sometimes does mean, however, that when our choices are limited, we may go looking elsewhere for answers. Today's doctors need to understand that when we feel backed into a corner and have our lives on the line, we are liable to do whatever needs to be done in order to help ourselves.

Imagine how you might feel if your doctor simply asked how he could support you. It would create tremendous rapport. It would also make you more willing to try Western medicine should alternative methods fail, instead of fearing an "I told you so" attitude.

Five little words—"How can we support you?"—can make a monumental difference. These words are like manna from heaven. They make a us feel heard and validated. They also encourage continuous open dialogue. Doesn't it make sense to know and understand what the patient is doing and perhaps even be surprised by a positive result?

———

It was hard for me to be on my own. I felt that my choice was between the traditional medical way and some other way that was poorly regarded. Although I talked to Jean Remmer from Hope & Cope about how I was feeling, there were only so many options she could offer me back then. Hope & Cope was the new kid on the block and had to be very careful about what they suggested outside the scope of traditional medicine, especially since they were hospital-based. Today, they offer many comprehensive and innovative programs. But at that time, I felt isolated and unsure of my choices. I had no one to talk to about nontraditional therapies and was lucky that I'd survived some very poor decisions. I hated that I was hiding what I was doing from my doctors. There were times when even making an attempt to bring up certain subjects for dis-cussion immediately led to an absolute "no." When someone is so close-minded, there is no point in further trying to have your voice heard. It made me sad, because I really needed to have dialogue with someone I trusted, even to have them explain to me why a certain direction might be the wrong one. In order to keep my sanity, I did what I needed to do, and I never discussed any of my "alternative" treatment choices with my doctors.

One of the many things I learned from having had cancer was the necessity for collaboration. We look to our doctors with the hope that they can fix us. In truth, I think that's asking too much. We would never have only one person build a house for us. It requires many trades coming together to achieve success. I believe that health is like that. Expecting one person to do everything is asking the impossible. It would take a lot of pressure off of both doctors and patients if cooperation between disciplines became commonplace.

In 2000, my husband became president of the Jewish General Hospital. It was a volunteer job (which took about thirty hours a week) and his way of giving back to an institution which had done so much for me. One of the oncologists met Jon in the hallway. After congratulating him on his new position, the doctor said he hoped Jon wasn't going to bring the witchcraft his wife practiced into the hospital with him. He was referring to my private practice, which incorporated various forms of complementary medicine along with traditional Western practices.

In 2004, I was invited by Dr. Walter Gotlieb to join the gynecology oncology tumor board as a natural health consultant. Dr. Gotlieb is the director of gynecologic oncology at the Segal Cancer Centre of the Jewish General Hospital, as well as director of surgical oncology at McGill University, where he is a professor in ob-gyn and oncology. He understood that simply focusing on the physical health of his patients was not enough. All components of whole person care must also be looked into. Each member of the team has an area of expertise. We work together to provide what the others might be missing in order to address the physical, psychological, and emotional needs of each patient.

There are lots of questions to ask. Does the patient want treatment that might interfere with their quality of life? How can we help them physically and emotionally as we remove body parts? What are the patient's religious or cultural beliefs? Can these beliefs help or even damage them during this very difficult time? Do we have the right to interfere with a patient's choice of death over major surgeries that leave them with bags instead of bladders and rectums? I remind the other members on the board that those who are leaving this world are as important as those who are entering it. We sometimes just need to remember to hold our patients' hands and allow them to feel partnered in their journeys. We must treat one another with respect and dignity. We are complex human beings who are often frightened and fragile. We all deserve to be handled with gentleness, kindness, and empathy

———

· *working together* ·

UNLESS DOCTORS LEARN to listen in a nonjudgmental manner, they will never really know what goes on with their patients behind closed doors. Whether we have their approval or not, we will try different things if there is a chance we think they might help us. Sometimes logic and good sense get thrown out the window when we are fighting for our lives! Why would we share our thought processes with doctors if all we get from them is disapproval? The catch is that our choices could not only be potentially damaging to us physically but frustrating to a doctor who might not be able to effectively evaluate our progress if he does not know what we are doing.

Dr. Herbert Benson is a cardiologist and the founder of the Institute for Mind Body Medicine at Massachusetts General Hospital in Boston. He wrote a book entitled *Timeless Healing: The Power and Biology of Belief,* in which he noted how potent a tool belief can be. He inferred that doctors' beliefs influence their patients. He felt it was extremely difficult for patients to actualize (make real) healing and recovery that their doctor didn't believe to be possible.

We need our doctors to walk alongside us. It is very hard to navigate illness and treatment alone. Patients and doctors need to become a team. Imagine specialists from all modalities working together to achieve our best possible outcome. We would feel supported not just physically but also mentally, emotionally, and spiritually.

———

WHEN I FINISHED three months of 714X injections, I went back to the lab in Rock Forest to find out whether there were any notable changes in my blood. I was thrilled! I could see progress before my very own eyes. My blood cells, which had looked thick and stuck together after the first test, appeared to be flowing freely and easily. A lot of what looked like debris from the cancer cells seemed to be gone. Whether this contributed to a placebo effect, I will never know. Frankly, I don't even care. This was the first time I could actually monitor my progress, and I was on cloud nine. By the end of the nine months, I was done. My blood results were excellent. I felt that my internal environment was beginning to support health and well-being. I felt empowered.

I worked hard on myself during the next few years, and as my strength came back, I reveled in how well I was able to function with just one lung. It was a far cry from how I initially felt. Every movement had been difficult then, and each breath was labored. I used to be embarrassed when I heard how loudly I breathed when exercising. Sometime the noise was deafening to me, and I felt ashamed. In time, I grew stronger, and the noises emanating from within me were not so bothersome.

A few years after lung surgery, Jon and I managed to bike up mountains in Italy and hike the trails in Tucson, Arizona. I would tell everyone around me not to worry, that I just breathed more heavily than they did because I had only one lung. They had two, so the sound was more muffled. It really is amazing how we eventually manage to move beyond our personal limitations. I remember climbing the Grand Canyon with Jon, Linda, and Stephen. I may have huffed and puffed my way up, but I was ahead of our little group by forty-five minutes. I was tickled pink! I was so grateful to be able to function reasonably well again and take pleasure in so many of the things I had enjoyed before.

Even today, nineteen years after my lung was removed, I still sound like I am making a supreme effort when exercising. Somehow, however, I have gotten used to it. At times, I do not even hear myself anymore. I have just as much capacity as anyone else and do whatever is within my ability to keep this lung strong and healthy.

(12)

SO MUCH
TO LEARN

IT WAS 1998, and my home life was really starting to feel peaceful. I felt safe inside my skin, and the threat of cancer returning rarely entered my thoughts. I guess I was too busy living my life to waste my energy going to a place I had already visited twice. If that was what the future had in store for me, I was not going to go there before I absolutely had to. The girls were growing nicely. Perhaps I had not given them as much time as I might have if I had not gotten sick, but they were not complaining. The two older ones were already in university and well on their way toward independence. Katherine was becoming a world traveler like her father, and Jacqueline was in acupuncture school. They seemed to be launched, but I felt that Ali wasn't quite there. Although we often sat and talked, she was the one I knew the least. I was so busy fighting for my life that I often felt that Ali was raised by her sisters. To this day, I am so grateful that she grew into an incredible strong, passionate, and loving woman.

As parents we try our best to minimize our children's suffering. We hope that they will learn from our life lessons. Kids, however, seem to need to experience everything firsthand. My two older girls smoked, and it drove me crazy. It was next to impossible for me not to judge their actions. I could not believe that after watching me struggle for breath, they even dared to pick up a cigarette. Perhaps it was a form of rebellion. Part of me hated them for doing it. I wanted to shake them in the hope of knocking some sense into them.

One evening, I was sitting with Jon in the den, talking about this frustration. Ali had just turned seventeen. I told him I was glad at least one of our children had not picked up that filthy habit. I was met with silence. Clearly, Jon knew something I did not. At that moment, Ali walked into the house and bounded up the stairs. She saw from the look in my eyes that I was upset. After I asked her point blank if she smoked, she burst into tears and told me it was so unfair that I found out while she was in the process of quitting.

I quickly left the room. Both she and Jon were smart enough not to follow me into my bedroom. I got undressed, washed my face, and brushed my teeth. I then buried myself under the blankets and cried for what felt like forever. I had felt so guilty for putting my family through so many hardships. I had hoped that I had not given them "bad genes," setting them up for a life filled with health challenges. I realized in that moment that I was not responsible for the outcome of their lives. As much as I might care for them, they were going to have to be the ones responsible for the consequences of their actions. The illusion I had of being able to protect them melted away like a block of ice under a hot summer sun. There was no way I could save them from pain and anguish. I could barely save myself. It was up to them to pick and choose how they were going to live their lives. I was not a smoker, and cancer still found its way to settle in my lung. If that was going to become their reality, there was little I could do about it. It was time to let go of the guilt I had held inside for so long. It was now up to them to chart the course of their lives. The only life I seemed to have partial control of was my own. I was going to do the very best I could to walk my talk. My hope was that they would make good decisions.

The next morning, Ali said she had a cold and decided to stay home from school. Part of me wondered if, after the events of the previous evening, she needed to make sure that I was not angry or disappointed in her.

The weather that day was absolutely frigid. Winter still had its hold on us even though it was mid-March. My dog, Scruffy, hated the bitter cold. I decided to let her out on the back balcony to do her business so that her little paws wouldn't get sore from the ice and salt that coated the sidewalks. Just as I let her out, a large icicle fell from the roof and pinned her leg to the ground. She let out a sickening yelp, and I ran outside barefoot to pick her up. Her leg was almost completely severed. I wrapped her in a blanket and got Ali to hold her while I drove to the animal hospital. Scruffy was sedated immediately, and the doctors needed her to rest a few days before they would be able to operate on her. They advised me not to visit, as she would get excited when she saw me and they needed her to remain quiet. I never got to see her again.

It was early Saturday morning and we were in the country when Jon got the phone call. My husband awakened me with the news. Scruffy had survived the operation but died from the shock. I yelled and screamed, throwing pillows at him as though it was somehow his fault. My sweet little dog—I could not believe she was gone. She had been mine from the start. My girls had wanted a larger dog, but Scruffy made her way into my heart the moment I saw her. I was devastated and cried the entire day, mourning her loss. I imagined holding her in my arms and rocking her gently as I said good-bye. She had been by my side from the moment I rescued her from the animal shelter, just before I was diagnosed with colon cancer. I think it was really Scruffy who rescued me with her unconditional love, rather than the other way around. As I sat there and envisioned rocking her, I decided she had left me knowing I was now well and it was her time to go off and help somebody else.

The way we choose to think can make living easier or more difficult. I did not deny the fact that Scruffy died. I put a different spin on it to make living with what had happened bearable. Through her death, she left me with one final gift: the belief that I really was healthy and well.

I WANTED TO continue learning as much as I could about the mind-body connection. So once again, I went back to school. This time, I decided to study neuro-linguistic programming (NLP). NLP involves a variety of techniques to help you overcome personal obstacles and realize your goals. It is a way of training your mind to see things differently and create a more positive attitude toward life. Tad James was my teacher. He graduated with a master's degree in mass communication and in 1988 wrote a book called *Time Line Therapy and the Basis of Personality*. I knew that incorporating some of his communication skills into my life would not only help me become a better therapist but also enable me to handle some of my difficult personal relationships more effectively.

The intention of Tad's work was to help people transform their behaviors in order to live better lives. For me, NLP is simply the study of how we take in the information that exists out in the world and use that information to formulate our ideas, beliefs, and core values. The question is, "Do these ideas, beliefs, and values serve me well, or do they not, and if not, what can I do about it?" By using some of these techniques, I was able to shift, or reframe, some of my limiting beliefs and live a happier, more fulfilled life. I looked at NLP as a way of growing and continuously making changes. I had done it unconsciously when my dog died. As I practiced these techniques over and over again, they became second nature to me. The Vietnamese Buddhist monk Thich Nhat Hanh once said, "If at first you don't believe it, fake it. Eventually you will come to believe it." We need to keep repeating to ourselves those thoughts and ideas that are good for us so that we can live well, irrespective of our circumstances.

· neuro-linguistic programming ·

AN EXAMPLE OF NLP in action might be the way your gut tightens up when you're speaking to someone who upsets you. Once you recognize the fact that you are holding tension in your belly, you can do what is called a pattern interrupt (changing a habitual reaction). You can take a deep breath and release it slowly, imagining all the tension evaporating through the pores on your skin. Then you can imagine warmth filling your body, making you feel so good that it brings a smile to your face. It is very hard to be upset and calm at the same time. With a mere breath, you have changed the state of your being and will be better able to handle a difficult situation. By simply recognizing the fact that you are holding tension in your belly, you are already on the road to rectifying the situation. The more we restrict an area, the greater chance we have of feeling awful. I often ask my clients to clench their fists really tightly. After a few minutes, their fingers change color. You can easily see that the blood is not flowing to their hands. Imagine what is happening inside our bodies when we hold on to that tension for a long time. How great would it be if we could get to the tension before the tension gets to us?

Another technique of NLP is reframing (changing the way you view a situation). It could be as simple as imagining a treatment being good for you as opposed to thinking that it will make you sick. Should you choose to undergo chemotherapy, it might serve you better to think of it as the magic elixir instead of a toxic poison. Believing the medicine knows exactly how to get to all the corners of your body, scouting out and killing any potential cancer cells, can make the treatments so much easier to take. How we choose to think about different situations helps to create what becomes our reality. Yes! It *is* true! It's all in our heads!

————

Some people think NLP is a form of manipulation. It probably could be, if used incorrectly. Many psychologists study NLP today knowing that it could be a valuable tool for helping their clients. It is an incredible field with the potential of opening many doors. It helped me gain better control in all areas of communication. I learned to create stories around difficult situations that allowed me to let go of the emotional pain I had kept locked up inside. Once, when I was giving a lecture, someone from the audience asked me how they could deal with a difficult family member. This subject had been my Achilles heel for a long time. I explained to my audience what I had done in this situation. I asked them to see only the mouth of the person they were having trouble with, opening and closing rapidly (a bit like a baby bird's does). I then suggested that they imagine pressing a mute button so that they had a comical picture of the mouth in action without any audible sound. I asked them to imagine shrinking that image down to the size of a postage stamp and placing it in their back pocket, exactly where it belonged. I patted my rear end when I said it, and everyone had a good laugh. At the end of the lecture, my mother asked me if I ever did that to her. "Only when I need to," I replied. She did not think that was very funny.

NLP was good for me because it gave me a formula that I could apply to many areas of my life. The master's-level course took place in Hawaii. We studied day and night for more than a month, with just a few days off to relax. During one of our off times, I booked a session with a kahuna, a Hawaiian healer. I wasn't sure what I expected, but after two cancers, I figured that I could use as much healing as I could get. Mostly, I was curious to see how he worked. I went to see him with one of the teachers I really trusted from my course. There was no way I was doing any of this alone again. She had seen him once before on a personal level and thought that we might be a good fit.

What I am about to share will probably sound crazy, and I can say that if it did not happen to me, as open as I am to different approaches, I probably would not have believed it.

We arrived in the room, and this man met us with a huge smile and sparkling face. There was no way I could determine his age. He could have been sixty or ninety. There was something about him that had the youthfulness of the young and the sage wisdom of the aged. He twinkled at me like my father did, and I felt peaceful and safe right away. The healer never said a word to me in English. He did not have to. After he muttered a few incantations in a language I did not understand, his gestures led me to understand that he wanted to put his hands on my chest, where the large scar from the lung cancer surgery was. Shyly, I nodded. Lo and behold, right before my eyes a thick line that looked like my scar appeared on his hands and arms. When I looked down at my chest, all that remained was a very thin, pencil-like scar you could barely see. I looked up into his eyes, which glistened like shiny stars as he smiled and bowed to me. I did not need words. Those eyes told me all I needed to know. I was all right.

When I returned to Montreal, my husband was visibly shaken when he saw the change in the scar. He used to joke about my explorations of alternative therapies, saying things like, "In another century, you would have been burned at the stake." After this experience, even Jon, with his scientific A-type personality, was becoming a believer. "See?" I told him. "There is so much out there that we don't know and will probably never understand. It affirms my belief that there really is magic in the world."

I will never be able to explain what happened. All I know is that my experiences have helped me become less quick to judge. I listen with more than my ears, and I have learned to see with more than my eyes. Events have been documented from the beginning of time that appear to have little scientific basis. Rather than attempting to disprove these events, I simply allow myself to marvel at their possibility. They fill me with hope for a better tomorrow and remind me daily of how much I need to learn.

ANOTHER AMAZING PHENOMENON happened when I went to a conference in Palm Desert called "Clinical Applications of Behavioral Medicine." In the United States, health care is big business. It behooves the doctors to know what their patients want, and offer it to them. These conferences have reputable speakers from many fields, all involving mind-body medicine. They also offer both pre- and post-conference workshops exploring various disciplines. One of the workshops was a course on qigong.

I had begun studying qigong at the Natural Health Consultants Institute. Part of traditional Chinese medicine, qigong is a form of exercise and movement intended to enhance inner healing by opening up the energy channels in the body. This allows for good flow of blood and *qi* (life force). It helps balance the body, and a balanced body is a healthy body. Many qigong masters practice four to five hours a day to keep their energy strong and to supplement their reserves.

I took a three-day pre-conference workshop with one hundred other people (more than half of them medical doctors) and witnessed three spontaneous healings (unexpected healings or cures) during the time I was there. One man suffered from cellulitis in his leg. Cellulitis is a bacterial infection between the skin and the muscle. It looks like cellulite, strangely bumpy but quite red and angry-looking. Another woman had such badly twisted hands from arthritis that she couldn't even hold a pencil. By the time the workshop came to a close, the man's skin was much less red, and all of the bumps were gone. His leg looked as smooth as a baby's. The woman was able to straighten out her hand, and for the first time in a long while, she was able to lift a pitcher of water and pour herself a drink. They were beyond elated. Both were essentially healed after three days.

Even I might have been skeptical if the third healing hadn't been mine. Luke Chan was our teacher and qigong master. The form we practiced was called Chi-Lel Qigong, a type of group healing. On the third day, he asked me whether he could put his hands on my chest. First the kahuna healer had asked for permission to touch my chest, and now the qigong master. My chest seemed to be calling out for attention. After I gave him permission, he placed his hand gently on my sternum, the bone between the lungs. The pain I immediately felt was so searing, that tears streamed down my face. I thought my chest wall was going to explode. But from that moment on I never wheezed or whistled again when I spoke.

When I returned to Montreal, my pulmonologist told me that a shift had occurred in my thoracic cavity that totally freaked him out. I implored him to tell my story to other patients who were having a tough time dealing with issues surrounding lung cancer. Unfortunately, he told me that he could not. I was already an enigma to him. The lung that was removed had three lobes in it, whereas the left lung has only two. I had expanded my left lung, which had been forty-five percent of my breathing capacity from birth, to more than eighty-five percent, with a saturation rate (which measures how well oxygenated your blood is) of almost one hundred percent. My doctor explained that a person born with one lung might be expected to see those results, but for someone in their forties, it was beyond anything he could have ever imagined possible. He said that if he ever got sick, it was me he was coming to see. He also told me that if another doctor had told him of my success, he would have found it very difficult to believe. I said I was glad that no one had ever told me I couldn't do it. I also said that he was limiting his patients by what *he* believed to be possible.

To this day, I do not understand why doctors do not try to explore these unexplainable successes to see exactly what people have done to exhibit such remarkable recoveries. Are they so fearful of touching upon other aspects of well-being that go beyond a traditional medical scope? Or are they simply limited by the overwhelming burdens already placed upon them?

We need to continue to be curious and open to possibilities. We have to remember that we can't do this alone. Health is multifaceted and requires so many disciplines.

―――

· *keeping an open mind* ·

ARE WE SO arrogant as to believe that we have all the answers? Has our statistical data shown such vast improvements with the methods we are presently using? Are we so sure of ourselves in the West that we think no other system of medicine can possibly work? We may not understand them all, but many have been around for a very long time.

I know of one patient who abandoned Western medicine in favor of a traditional Hindu Ayurvedic approach. She was born in India and believed that this was the best choice for her, culturally and spiritually. Her decision was extremely upsetting for her Western-trained doctors, who believed that she might succumb to the cancer faster without chemotherapy. Perhaps the medicines she wanted to try could put her cancer in remission. Perhaps her beliefs would activate a placebo response that could move her toward health and well-being. We will never know for sure. Although none of us are certain of the future, at the moment she is still doing well. There are many reports of spontaneous remissions without any scientific basis behind them.

Many native cultures throughout the world have used all kinds of natural medicines from trees and flowers for centuries, treating certain cancers and illnesses that Western medicine is only now trying to run trials on, for billions of dollars. When you are dying and all the traditional drugs you have tried show no promise, is there anything wrong with trying other healing remedies and therapies that seem to have worked in other cultures? I have witnessed firsthand in the Amazon jungle, Costa Rica, and Guatemala how generations of healers were taught by the medicine man or family members to successfully deal with numerous illnesses using the flora and fauna in their midst.

Understand that I am not endorsing any one thing in particular; I am simply saying that closing the doors to any possibility is not an optimal approach. I have never believed that the world exists in only black and white. There will always be things we do not understand. That does not necessarily make them dangerous or wrong.

———

When I was attending the Natural Health Consultants Institute, we had a three-day workshop held in the Eastern Townships. One of the exercises was a form of what is called "rebirthing." Although it seemed quite contrived at the time, it was interesting to experience. We formed two rows facing each other and then sat down, crossing our legs over one another. Each person had a turn crawling or wiggling through a sea of legs. Some screamed, some cried, some whimpered, and yet each person was so excited that they had done it. They made it through without any help and felt a tremendous sense of accomplishment in the process.

It seemed to be the pattern in the school that I was always selected last for each exercise. I had quietly joked with Jon that this was a school of epiphanies left, right, and center. It felt like many who were enrolled at the school went there simply for three or four years of intense therapy. This time, however, I was the one having an epiphany. As I pushed through the sea of legs (and I swear they made it really difficult for me on purpose), I decided to lie there quietly and wait. Something inside me refused to struggle and fight. I had done so much of that in the past. It was time to simply allow. Finally, after about five to ten minutes, I heard a voice (someone playing midwife) ask if I needed help. I said yes and was pulled out effortlessly.

When asked to share my experience, I beamed, saying that it was such a pleasure to know that I never had to do it alone again. Been there, done that. John Harricharan's book title came to mind: *When You Can Walk on Water, Take the Boat*. There is so much help out there just waiting to be accessed. My teacher smiled at me, not needing to say a word.

· *accepting help* ·

HELP MEANS RENDERING assistance, nothing more. It doesn't mean taking over the job of another person. I think illness is often a harsh reminder that things have changed and we may not be able to do as much as we did before. We need to adjust how we feel about accepting help, because all of us can use it from time to time. Accepting help does not mean that we have no capacity to do something ourselves. It simply means that we can share the task.

Help often comes to us in unconventional ways. Sometimes, in the face of adversity, we are forced to move in a direction we never expected to go. I occasionally wonder what my life might have been like without all the physical and emotional suffering I experienced. I have grown up and survived in spite of it all, and I am still in awe of my personal resilience. I have to admit, though, that I don't think I could have made it without the tremendous support I had from so many who may never even know the roles they played in my life.

————

I ONCE ATTENDED a conference where Dr. Rachel Naomi Remen was a guest speaker. At the time, she was the medical director of the Commonweal Cancer Help Program, an organization started by a man named Michael Lerner to investigate various alternative and complementary treatments for cancer. Dr. Remen told us a story about a young man who was very ill with Crohn's disease. He was morose, in constant pain, and had suicidal thoughts. Although he did not have cancer, she was willing to see if she could help him feel better. He was unable to talk to anyone about what he was feeling and refused all forms of help. He was getting sicker and sicker by the day, but she refused to give up on him. One day, he told her that he had had a dream in which he saw a baby being stabbed in the belly with a knife. At first, he was quite shocked by the violence, but it was what happened afterwards that was remarkable. Once the baby was stabbed, the young man watched, in what appeared to be time-lapse photography, the baby grow. First, he grew into a toddler, then a child, then an adolescent, and finally into a man. The bigger he grew, the smaller the knife appeared to be. The ache became less noticeable as well.

Dr. Remen told him that all of us suffer anguish, and part of the human experience is the notion that we are all born flawed. She said that it is only through these flaws that spirit can enter. He started to understand that his body was not his enemy, something he needed to continuously fight against. He began to open up and express his emotions and realized that he did not have to do it alone. Finally, he was at peace, and he slowly began to heal.

I was so moved by this story that I had to run out of the conference room, and I found myself crying uncontrollably. "It is through these flaws that spirit can enter" was all I could hear. I had tried for so long to accept the way my abdomen looked. I had been able to change my thinking and perspective on so many things. Why was accepting my physical appearance such a struggle? I had hated the mess that was my belly. It had so many scars and lumps and bumps. I had to continually adjust my clothing so that the world would never know I had this secret imperfection. Not a day went by when I did not think about this belly of mine. This inability to accept my physical appearance led me to a plastic surgeon ten years after the colon cancer surgery. I booked reconstructive surgery to clean up the mess, but cancelled when an osteopath told me "not to be so superficial with something so deep." "Don't stir the pot," he said. "You might activate something that is sleeping." I listened to him out of fear and accepted the fact that it was far better to have the scars than not to have my life.

It's hard for another person to understand how profound Dr. Remen's words were for me. Gifts don't always come packaged in the way we might expect. My husband had tried to reassure me for ten years how beautiful I was and how the scars did not affect him at all. The problem was that they were not his scars; they were mine. If acceptance doesn't come from within, reassurance has a short shelf life. In that moment, I understood that my belly was my friend and found myself rubbing and soothing it continually, like a pregnant woman.

―――――

· *support* ·

Reach, reach out and take my hand.
Let me be there for you as spirit,
Let me be there for you as friend.
The pain we experience is so hard to bear alone.
A kindness, a gesture, an ear that listens
Is more than enough to open the door
To know that loneliness doesn't have to feel so lonely.
This experience of fear, of vulnerability,
Strips away the facade we think protects us.
Is the tree less beautiful without any leaves?
How freeing it must be to walk unmasked,
Stripped of the window dressings we use on a regular basis,
Naked in our honesty.
A diagnosis of cancer fracturing all we thought solid,
All lost in an abyss of emptiness,
Nothing to hang on to except one another.
So reach, reach out and take my hand,
Allow me to see you as you are,
The perfection of the imperfection.
I cannot take away your experience.
I cannot shield you from your pain.
But if you let me carry you, and hold you in my arms,
Perhaps the burden of all that you face
Mightn't feel so heavy after all.

(13)

COMPLICATIONS

BEFORE THE COLON resection, I had textbook bowel movements. Don't laugh; this was really a big deal. So many people in my family dealt with constipation issues that we could have owned a plum orchard for all the prunes we seemed to ingest. My dad and I could proudly proclaim that going to the bathroom had never been a problem for either of us.

Everything changed after the colon cancer surgery. My normal of the past was not the normal of the present. I often had feelings of fullness (like when you have eaten way too much and think you are going to burst). My three-times-a-day habit of going to the bathroom had changed to sometimes going only once every three days. I could deal with these changes, especially since they were by-products of a surgery that had saved my life. But then things went from bad to worse. I started getting both small and large bowel obstructions following the surgery to remove my ovary. These obstructions were excruciatingly painful. I guess the body really doesn't like being disturbed, and mine had been invaded far too many times. I was riddled with scar tissue.

Bowel adhesions (scar tissue) can create kinks (twists or curves), and just like a garden hose when pinched, they limit or completely block the flow of waste products. These adhesions form whenever there is inflammation. They can also form at surgical sites. The body tries to heal itself by creating a kind of internal scab, which protects the wound. My doctors felt that this was what was happening to me. According to them, there was not much that could be done. Carol-Ann told me that she really did not want to go into my belly again unless she had absolutely no choice. She led me to believe that my insides were a real mess and she did not want to make matters worse (since each intervention can create even more scar tissue).

Initially, the obstructions forced me to be hospitalized only once a year. The flurry of activity around me each time was impressive. The doctors were constantly checking for cancer. I guess since I'd had it twice, they expected it to show up again. I knew without question that these obstructions had nothing to do with cancer. It was the medical team and my family that needed to be reassured, not me.

There was only one time following the second cancer that I ever thought, "Oh no, here we go again," and worried that the ugly little monster might rear its head once again. It was a Friday afternoon. Never go and see your doctor on a Friday afternoon. If something is uncertain, you spend the weekend suffering before anything can be done. I went to my family doctor for a routine physical examination. She felt an enlarged lymph node on the right side, where I'd had the lung removed. It was just under my breast. She wanted me to see a breast surgeon to rule out the possibility of cancer. I was stunned. "You have to be kidding," I thought. "This cannot be happening again."

I left her office and walked to the nearest phone. For whatever reason, perhaps because I started crying uncontrollably and the receptionist felt sorry for me, I got an appointment with the surgeon for the following Monday. Then I went home in a daze, packed up the car, and headed to the country with my husband (sounds like a pattern, huh?). This time, I was not so cool. I insisted on driving, since I hate Jon's driving (I swear, I never know how he makes it anywhere without me!). I cried so hard that I could have used a pair of windshield wipers for my eyes. Once again, there was Jon, scared but not knowing how to help me. I was inconsolable. "How could God be so cruel?" I asked him. "Not once or twice, but three times?" I felt that this was more than I could bear. The memories of everything I had been through, all I had suffered, came back in a flurry. All of my strength and determination disappeared. I wasn't sure I could survive another test. Jon was smart enough not to say a word. Sometimes, when things are really bad, words are not helpful. Just knowing that someone is there is enough. In the state I was in, I am sure I would have taken anything the wrong way that came out of his mouth.

Once inside the house, I ran upstairs, brushed my teeth, washed my face, and told Jon I was going to bed. He asked if I wanted him to make me dinner. I said no, I had no appetite. Although it was barely 6:30 p.m., he knew better than to argue with me. I told him that I needed to be alone and that I was going to pray. I needed to find my footing and knew that I could do so if I immersed myself in a quiet, sacred space. If I could calm myself down, I might have half a chance to create an action plan. I reminded myself of the time I was celebrating my first anniversary post–colon cancer. I was in Florida with my parents, while Jon remained home in Montreal. Just as I was making a toast to being alive, my husband received a call from the hospital saying that my tumor marker (an indicator showing potential cancer activity) had gone up. My oncologist wanted me to return from holidays and come into the hospital for a full evaluation. Jon refused to tell me, suffering alone with the news of a potential recurrence. He figured that should the cancer be back, one more week would not make a difference. He wanted me to enjoy my celebration with my parents. In the end, I did not have a recurrence, and the elevation in the tumor marker turned out to be a false positive.

As I lay in bed, I hoped that perhaps this too would be nothing. Talking to God was what I needed for my sanity. From about 7 p.m. until 5 a.m., I prayed and repeated a mantra: "I am strong, I am healthy, I am safe, and God is with me." Finally, I fell into a deep and peaceful sleep. I woke up around noon, sat down, and wrote about fear. I went downstairs to find Jon and was eerily peaceful. I was completely calm and knew that, without question, I didn't have cancer. I passed the weekend quietly at the cottage, choosing to cocoon.

——

· *fear* ·

First you hear the words,
"We need to check this out, don't worry."
Innocuous in themselves, these words offer no
        answers nor hold any promise.
Stated as if matter of fact,
Like you were verifying the air pressure of a tire.
"We need to check this out, don't worry."
Words, simple words,
And yet, the power they possess is undeniable.
The potential story they house life-altering.

"Don't worry." What a joke!
How can anyone have the audacity to say that?
Just because I appear strong.
Just because I always manage to handle adversity.
Just because not one but two kinds of cancer didn't kill me.
Just because, in spite of it all, I basically happen
      to remain optimistic
Doesn't mean that at times it is not excruciatingly painful to be me.
I shift between letting myself feel and being detached.
I can sense my energy field closing in around me,
Doing what it can to protect me as if I were a sacred flower.
This is an old pattern, a tool I have used in the past.
It doesn't work for me any longer.
What I need now is the exact opposite.
If I could become expansive . . .
Perhaps I wouldn't feel the gripping in my throat
      choking off my every breath.
If I could become expansive . . .
Perhaps the pinpointed deep ache in my chest
Would allow my heart to beat more freely.
If I could become expansive . . .
I might imagine my belly opening
Breaking free from the cocooned beliefs that
      no longer serve me well.
I need to break the shackles that bind me.
I need to explode the fear into tiny droplets of water
That dissolve into the expanse of the endless sea.
I need to remember the hope, the familiar light, the
      potential that is mine!
My heartbeat begins to slow.
My armpits cease their endless sweat.

My belly finds its breath.
My soul once again timidly steps forward,
Willing, always willing, to hold my hand and take me home.

———

Monday came, and the doctor told me that the lymph node was enlarged because of all the bug bites I had gotten the weekend before in the country. My body was simply doing what it needed to do in order to keep me healthy. He was very impressed that my doctor had even noticed the node. He said that she had been remarkable in her attentiveness.

And there I was, safe once again. My concept of God intact, my beliefs reaffirmed. It is amazing how we can go from sanity to insanity and back to sanity in such a short period of time. We are capable of pushing through so much and still coming out the other side. We will all go through difficult times like this.

Some people ask me how it is possible to learn to trust their bodies over and over again, when every ache or pain seems to rain terror upon their soul. I don't really have an answer for them. Time and a variety of scares that turned out to be all right, and a lot of self-talk, helped me find peace within myself. So although my doctors kept me busy with every test known to man each time I had a partial bowel obstruction, I knew that I was all right. People, however, can die from many things other than cancer.

THE BOWEL OBSTRUCTIONS were becoming more than an occasional hiccup. They started interfering with my quality of life. It was 2004, ten years since the first time I had experienced one. I had hoped that they would magically disappear,

but instead they were becoming more frequent. I found it difficult to express the fear, pain, and frustration that surrounded
each episode. I didn't have cancer after all, so did I have the
right to complain? Was an episode every three or four months
so hard to bear? I tried to convince myself that I could handle
it but was starting to unravel. Rubin Becker had just become
my family doctor. He reminded me that he had met me when I
was in intensive care having just had a lung removed. As with
so many other memories, I had no recollection of meeting
him before. I was grateful to have such a kind and empathetic
doctor there for me. Our experiences drew us closer and our
families became fast friends. I do not think he had any idea
what he was getting into when he took me on as a patient.

Jon still dreamed about traveling the world, but I told him
that remote, exotic places where they did not speak English
were out for me. I no longer felt secure traveling far away from
home. As a result, after a lot of discussion, Jon and I thought
that Ireland might be a good place for us to go on a vacation. We
both love getting away from the hustle and bustle of city life,
and the idea of exploring the countryside made us happy. The
coastlines, rolling hills, and cascading waterfalls in Ireland are
exquisite. I discovered many excellent teaching hospitals in
the areas we were going to visit, should I need them. Can you
imagine that my vacations were now determined by where I
could find good medical care? I felt about a hundred years old.

We were having a wonderful time together, walking the
streets of Dublin, when I started to feel unwell. I was getting
pains in my stomach that seemed to make my entire abdomen
sore. My pants began to feel tighter as my abdomen started
to swell. I thought that I might be hungry, since many hours
had passed since my last meal and I am the kind of person who

needs to eat frequently. I am sometimes so excited by what I am doing that I don't notice I am hungry until I start to have a belly ache. We went to a restaurant to eat, but it was too late. I could barely touch my food. I sat there for what felt like an eternity, sweating profusely from the spasms in my gut. Eventually, I told Jon that I had to get out of there, as I was going to throw up. He paid the bill quickly and held my arm as we walked in the cool evening air.

For a moment, I felt better, and then an unbearable pain overtook me. I could not breathe. Jon told me that my eyes rolled into the back of my head, and I simply dropped like a dead weight in the middle of the street. He was certain that I had just died before his very eyes. He grabbed me by the shoulder, tearing the tissue that holds the bones in place, ensuring that I did not smash my head on the pavement. His quick actions probably saved my life. When I regained consciousness, the ambulance technician told me that my heart had stopped. I wondered: Can a pain be so horrible that rather than having to bear it, the body just decides to stop? The fact that my heart had stopped fascinated me. Nothing hurt any longer in those last moments. I thought I had fallen delicately like a leaf. Jon had a different impression; he had feared that this was my final exit. My father had recently died, and I thought a lot about him when I was in the ambulance. He had seemed so peaceful in those last moments. Did he feel what I had just experienced?

Jon was beside himself. He was visibly shaken. He sat beside me in the hospital, holding my hand and stroking my arm for hours. The doctors and nurses were amazing. I was taken care of immediately and probably given enough morphine to subdue an elephant. While waiting for blood tests and scans, I asked Jon for a pen and paper and wrote down my thoughts on death. As soon as I finished writing, I passed out and slept deeply. Once again, the partial obstruction reversed itself, and I left the hospital about eight hours later, exhausted and armed with pain medication. Jon took me to the hotel, where I slept for the remainder of the day while he went shopping. After all, what did I want him to do? Sit and look at me while I slept? The next morning, our guide had to stop the car half a dozen times while I threw up the effects of the morphine. I was a trooper and within a couple of days was back to myself, a few pounds lighter but none the worse for wear. Although it was very frightening to be so far away from home and the safety of my doctors, I received excellent medical care and will forever be indebted to the people of Ireland.

———

· *death* ·

Death, are you there?
What do you want?
I am trying to avoid you
But you seem better at the hunt.
Please go elsewhere and leave me alone.
I need my time to weep and my time to mourn.
You watch me like a panther
Hungry for its meal
Pacing back and forth, oh so surreal.
Are you waiting for me to surrender?
Into what I do not know?
To fall into nothingness
Can be a fearful place to go.
My body may be weak and appear easy game,

But my spirit is strong, forever to remain
A part of all that is.
Of this I am sure.
I am changing, I am shifting
Breaking free from constraint.
I am aching, I am stretching
As I prepare to meet my fate.
A freedom so pure
The nectar so sweet
The gift of forever, a blessing, a treat.
I am ready, I am calm
I am safe and content.
Breaking free from my skin
Is my only intent
As I step into freedom.

———

By the time 2005 arrived, I really did not want to travel anymore. I was obstructing more frequently. The anxiety of getting sick anywhere other than home left me in a panic. Jon was disappointed, but eventually he came around. I encouraged him to travel with friends or his kids to all the places I could not visit. He did, and even took Kassy to Thailand for a month. My guilt was eased, as I felt I was no longer holding him back from doing the things he loved. I am by nature a home-body, so this was not a huge personal sacrifice.

There was no question, however, of my not going to Vancouver. Jon and I had started going there together after we married. We skied the mountains in Whistler, him joyfully, me terror-stricken. Downhill skiing was his passion, but I had taken it up only out of love for him. I do not like speed, and it was exhausting to continually descend those huge hills. Cross-country skiing and snowshoeing are much more my style.

At various times, all my children lived in British Columbia. Alexandra graduated from high school with honors and chose to go to Vancouver for university. Kassy took some time off to travel after high school and then went to the University of Victoria. In time, both girls moved back to Montreal. But then Jacqueline moved to Vancouver, hoping to make a life for herself after completing her master's in acupuncture and Chinese medicine. There she met her husband, Andy, and started a family. As grandchildren started to come, it was so important for me to be a part of their lives. I put my fears aside and traveled there, comforted that I was still in Canada.

Jacqueline had a difficult pregnancy with Jonah and was on bed rest for thirty-two weeks. He arrived three weeks later, the cutest little peanut at just over five pounds. I told Jacqueline that I had a dream of him running across the airport as a toddler into my arms. When that indeed happened, I cried from pure joy. My original goal was to see my kids out of high school. Never at that time did I even dare to hope for more. Today I feel so blessed and grateful to have seven grandchildren. Each of them holds a special place in my heart, and I cherish them as if they were precious jewels.

I had obstructed a few times on previous trips to Vancouver and was thankful that one of Jackie's best friends, Debbie Rosenbaum, is a doctor. Although I did have someone to watch my back if I got into trouble there, I usually called her only once I was in the emergency department, wanting to be certain I really needed her before I called and disturbed her home life.

St. Paul's, the hospital where Debbie works, serves many homeless people and drug addicts. Whenever I got sick, I chose to go to that hospital so that she could look in on me and manage my care. Once, I was in so much pain from an obstruction that my body started to shake uncontrollably. The shaking and shivering made the doctors think that I was a drug addict in withdrawal. They refused to give me any drugs, thinking that I came to hospital in need of a fix. Although I wasn't an addict, boy oh boy, did I ever need a fix. Morphine seemed to be the only thing that relieved the pain from these obstructions, but the side effects were nasty. Nausea and vomiting were not unfamiliar to me, but constipation (one of the main side effects) was not helpful when blocked insides were the problem. It seemed to be the only thing that relieved the pain, and doctors could offer me no alternative. I was lucky, though, because it usually took only three or four doses of morphine to get the spasms under control. When they came, however, they were so strong that they took my breath away. One time, the pain was so intense that my blood pressure spiked to 220 over 120. That was alarmingly high, and the doctors were worried that I could suffer a stroke if they didn't get the pain under control quickly. There were no available beds in the ER, so they placed me on a gurney in front of the nurses' station. They administered morphine to me every twenty minutes until the pain was tolerable.

It's remarkable that each time I obstructed, I was surprised. There were warning symptoms, after all. A general feeling of malaise seemed to overtake me. I had backaches, felt very bloated, and was quite lethargic. Yet no matter how aware I seemed to be, there appeared to be nothing I could do to nip the pain in the bud before it got to me. I tried to think it away. I tried to breathe it away. Regardless of how much practice or training I had, I failed miserably. I could not seem to calm or relax my body during these episodes. I taught visualization, meditation, and stress management. I believed in it; why couldn't I do it for myself when I was in trouble? I always tell my clients to practice the techniques in the good times, because it is so much harder to have control under duress. Perhaps I just needed to accept that this was something beyond my control and stop beating myself up.

It was frustrating for everyone around me to watch me go through these episodes time and time again. I started resenting everyone's opinions. They couldn't possibly understand what I was going through, yet they seemed to speak with such authority. Food took on a life of its own and at times became the ugly bug-eyed monster. Some said that I was not eating enough fiber. Some said I was eating too much fiber. "Just go on liquids. Leave out all roughage. Only eat white bread. Only eat whole grain products." You could go crazy from all the advice. Yet nothing I tried seemed to work. I became afraid to eat—I associated it not with pleasure but with pain. It is a wonder that I did not develop a severe eating disorder during this time. I stayed close to home, didn't go out much, and did my best to simply make it through each day. I hated calling Rubin and complaining all the time. He hunted for solutions but basically came up empty. My colorectal surgeon tried to have me modify my diet, but that had no effect on the obstructions. I often reminded myself how much I had to be grateful for. Jacqueline had two beautiful children, Ali had just married Pat, Kassy was healthy and well, and I was madly in love with my husband. All the hardships we had experienced together seemed to only bring us closer.

IN 2007, I was in Vancouver for Jonah and Ali's birthdays. Jon had just suffered a serious ski accident in which he pulled all the muscles in his groin, tore the rotator cuff in his shoulder, and dislocated and fractured his shoulder. He needed to rest for a few days before traveling home, so that the swelling would subside. He was on so much pain medication that he was calmer and more relaxed than usual. Since Jon has trouble sitting still at the best of times, he insisted on going out for dinner and celebrating Ali's birthday a few days after the accident (my grandson's birthday passed with Jon stoned on morphine—I am not sure he even remembered being there!). I was happy to be with my kids and their husbands. Ali and Pat were going to be returning home to Montreal in a few months, and it was a treat for us to be together.

During dinner, I started to feel unwell. "Please, please don't make this night about me," I thought. I tried my best to wish the pain away, with little success. My body seemed to have a mind of its own, and it let me know that it was in control. I knew I was exhausted because I had slept little the few nights before, taking care of my husband, but there were no other warning signs. I could not even put a morsel of food in my mouth, and I just sat there, trying to make small talk, quite unsuccessfully. "Not again," I thought. All it took was one look from the kids to know that I had ruined the evening. They wanted to leave right away, but in accordance with my stoic nature, I refused and told them that this was important to me. I guess it was hard to argue with that logic. As soon as dinner was over (no one stayed for coffee), we gave Ali her twenty-sixth birthday present and went en masse to the hospital.

Debbie was out of town, so instead of going to St. Paul's, where I had become a regular visitor, we went to the closest hospital, which was Vancouver General. Once I was assessed and given morphine to make me more comfortable, a team of doctors came into the room to consult with us. They were worried. A CT scan showed that I was not only obstructed but also had four lesions on my spleen. The look on the girls' faces was morose. They were afraid to even glance my way. Thank God each of them had her husband by her side. Jon handled it much better, probably because he was on drugs. I, for some reason, was not the least bit worried. I knew that I was not completely out of touch with reality. I just felt that this was not cancer. I'd had so many scares in the past that turned out to be just that—scares. The doctors did not want to investigate further, as I had a medical team already working with me back in Montreal. They suggested I return home as soon as possible because they feared that the cancer had spread once again. My family supported me lovingly, but I could tell they were scared.

Jon and I returned home as quickly as we could make arrangements. It turned out that the spleen lesions had been noted from the first scan, when I was diagnosed in 1989 with colon cancer. They could have been there from birth. The important part was that they had never grown and were of no concern. My gut had been correct. I was no longer in fear of my body with respect to cancer; I just couldn't seem to get it to cooperate in stopping these obstructions.

Eventually, the obstruction reversed itself and life continued as usual. I thought I was going to Vancouver to help Jon after his accident, but I ended up once again being the focus of attention. As much as I may appreciate a certain amount of attention, I hate getting it because I am sick.

My daughters handled each obstruction episode really well (they sure had enough experience). They were upset, of course, but chose to live in the moment with me. They were able to comfort me without smothering me and still get on with their own lives. For them, not living in the same city as me had some benefits in this regard.

Jon handled my obstructions differently, probably because my situation affected him the most and was difficult for him to escape. He could not stand to see the pain I was in and often went to the doctors for counsel. No one seemed to have the answer. He stood by helpless, unable to stop my suffering. He kept a lot of his feelings inside, and when he did not know what to do, he buried himself in his work.

As parents, we always hope that our wisdom, guidance, and life experiences will impact our children. All of my girls chose to work, like me, in health care. After completing her postgraduate work in Chinese medicine and acupuncture, Jacqueline continued her studies in life coaching and is presently doing a master's degree in counseling. She lives in Vancouver with her husband, Andy, and their children, Jonah, Laylah, and Jude.

Katherine studied massage and body work, as well as integrative Eastern and Western nutrition, and then went to acupuncture school. She spent a lot of time in India, learning as much as she could to create a whole person integrative practice. She lives in Montreal with her husband, Martin, and their boys, Mikha and Izaya.

Ali became a behavioral analyst, creating programs for children with autism. She teaches therapists specific approaches and techniques for working with that population. She also lives in Montreal, with her husband, Pat, and their two children, Téa and Cole.

Their lives are rich and full. Each of them is unique and a star in my eyes. They are continuously learning (as is their mother), striving to become the best they can be. They are my biggest teachers. I feel blessed to have been able to watch each of them flourish (and by the way, no one smokes any longer).

(14)

IS THIS REALLY
MY LIFE?

WE BOUGHT A small house across the lane from Jacqueline in
Vancouver almost a year after Jonah was born. Jon had worked
in Vancouver in the past, and he opened an office there once
again. In all the years we had been married, the house was the
only thing I had ever asked Jon for. I am not a jewelry person,
and have no interest in fancy clothes or cars. I do know, however, that I need my personal space in which to thrive. The
ability to be close to my daughter and her family when I visited,
but still to have my own place, was one of the best gifts I have
ever received. It made me feel that my visits were not an impo-
sition on Jackie or her family. As a matter of fact, our den is now
an office where Jackie sees her clients. It was a win-win situation. I loved the idea of raising my blinds each morning and
within minutes getting a phone call from my daughter wishing me good morning. I had always wanted to be able to help
with her family. Because she lived so far away, she was often on
her own handling whatever crisis came her way. As a mother
of three, I knew they could happen at any moment. I also knew
that the only way my grandchildren would ever really know
me was if I visited often.

Unfortunately, my plans did not turn out the way I had hoped. Instead of being able to help her, I was the one who seemed to require all the attention. Visiting was supposed to be fun, but over the last few years I was so preoccupied with myself that I wasn't having any! I was now afraid to even go to Vancouver. Although I missed playing with my grand-children, when I was there I couldn't be present in the way I really wanted to be.

Even in Montreal, I realized how little I wanted to be alone with Ali's daughter. It broke my heart when Ali told me one day that I was not giving her daughter, Téa, the kind of attention I had given Jacqueline's kids. I love that little girl with all of my heart, and just the thought of not being there for her ripped through my gut. Ali didn't realize I was trying my best just to be present when I saw her. Since Téa's birth, I never felt com-pletely well. When I was not obstructing, I was functional, but that is a far cry from feeling good. Living without intense pain was one thing, but I forgot what it was like to feel anything other than pain. I did my best to function and hid my feelings about my situation, since there appeared to be little I could do about it.

I cried myself to sleep that night. Ali was right. My love for all my grandchildren was equal, but the time I spent with them alone was not. I adored this sweet little girl, but I was scared. Jon was away a lot and not around to help me. I was rarely alone with Jackie's kids for long. We were usually together, me playing with them while she cooked or ran short errands. If I babysat at night, they were only a phone call away. It was hard for me to admit that being left alone with Téa petrified me. What if I didn't feel well? What if I had an attack? When one of those came, it was so strong that I was unable to function. And they were starting to come out of nowhere, with little warning. If that happened, would I be able to take care of her properly? My health was affecting my ability to enjoy my grandchildren, and I felt ashamed and disappointed in myself. All I had ever wanted was to have these little beings close to me. It devastated me that I was not being the grandmother I had hoped I could be. When my children were young, I had been the sick mother. Would I be leaving behind a legacy of being the sick grandmother as well? Just the idea made me want to throw up.

It was spring 2007, and Jon worked hard convincing me to travel to Vancouver once again. He thought that seeing the kids would lift my spirits. Knowing that he would be skiing in Whistler, not far away, in case I got into trouble, gave me the security I needed to go. I was sitting in the car with my granddaughter Laylah, when all of a sudden I turned white. Sweat started to pour down my face, and my entire body became damp and clammy. Jackie had just left us for a few moments while she ran in for a quick visit with her doctor. As soon as she came back and took one look at my face, she knew I was in trouble. I told her that I just needed to lie down and rest for a while. She didn't believe me, got scared, and called her father, telling him to come back to the city immediately. Whistler is only about a ninety-minute drive from Vancouver. He left quickly and was back at our house within a couple of hours.

That evening, I found myself in the emergency room once again. I was becoming a regular visitor and already had a huge file there. This time I was given morphine straight away to ease the pain. When I provided the nurse with a routine urine sample, alarm bells went off. My urine was ruby red. It looked as though it was full of blood. I was given a wide spectrum of antibiotics along with the morphine. They were taking no chances.

Yes, I was obstructed, but the doctors feared that I had a severe urinary tract infection at the same time. The antibiotics managed to further weaken my colon, and as a result I developed *C. difficile*, a bacterial infection. It destroys all the good bacteria (flora) that live in the colon and keep us healthy. With this infection, patients often experience pain, severe diarrhea, dehydration, and fever. Sometimes it can lead to life-threatening inflammation of the colon.

I did not know that I had *C. difficile* when I left the hospital the next morning, because the culture to determine whether I had it can take a few days to show a positive result. It was difficult for me to know the difference between the pain I felt with an obstructed bowel and the pain from the infection. When I got back to our Vancouver home, I knew that something was very wrong. This was different from any other obstruction I'd had in the past. Usually, when the attack was over, it was over. Although the doctors had told me that the obstruction seemed to have resolved itself, I still felt awful. I crawled up the stairs to my bedroom, got into bed, and lay there, curled up in a fetal position. For the first time since having children, I was so ill that I could not even talk to any of them for four days. After everything they had already gone through, this unnerved them completely. It was one thing for them to know that I was sick—that they were used to—but to be completely cut off from any form of communication with me was a different story. Jacqueline came to check on me. She stood at the foot of my bed with tears in her eyes. I had to close mine to avoid being drawn into her emotional spiral. I had no energy. I felt as though I was a balloon, slowly leaking my vitality. I was literally disappearing. I was very placid, but that behavior in itself brought out a lot of insecurities within my kids. At the best of times, Jon does not like spending a lot of time on the telephone, and here he was with it practically glued to his ear as he tried to reassure our daughters.

It was tough to explain how I felt. This was different from anything I had ever experienced before. I still had no idea that I had *C. difficile*. I thought my body must have become so exhausted and depleted after all the trauma it had gone through that recovery this time was slow. I was so drained that all I could do was simply lie in my bed. I couldn't watch television or even listen to the radio. Time was of no consequence. It just passed as I felt my life force drain from my body. What a strange dichotomy: a bowel obstruction usually doesn't let anything pass through you, whereas *C. difficile* doesn't allow you to keep anything in. I experienced an internal war so violent, with such profuse vomiting, that I had no energy left to even take a sip of water. I lay in bed, moaning, curled up in a little ball. I was completely aware of what was happening, and in some perverse way, I found it quite fascinating. Since I was unable to change the situation, I just changed how I saw it. I didn't panic. I didn't fight it. I simply allowed it to be as it was. I felt myself melting like a piece of ice bathed by the sun. It reminded me of a client of mine who went from fighting death with everything she had to a calm, quiet, peaceful acceptance of her fate.

———

· *acceptance* ·

Death, are you knocking?
Can I open the door?
Will it be horrors that greet me?

Might I dare to explore?
I fear what awaits me;
I know not what to expect.
My jaw clenched in anguish,
I painfully reflect.
I lived a lifetime of structure
Of rules by the book
Never stopping to wonder, to see, or to look.
I lost out on what was;
It didn't fit into my view.
Oh, how I wish that I could start anew.
Now how can I live, knowing
That no matter what I do
The ending is near.
I haven't finished my work;
There is so much to be done.
Will I have a chance to undo
The tight webs I have spun?
I am brittle. I am dry. I am tight, almost done.
I am cracking, I am breaking
I am releasing to the sun.
Please come and get me as I dissolve on the grass,
As I break into a million pieces like beautiful sacred glass
That reflects a prism, a myriad of colors.
The rainbows I see dance like Tinkerbells as they flutter.
I can breathe, I can move, I expand in the air.
I am growing, I am dancing with grace and with flare.
No longer am I burdened by my structure or my ways;
I explode into freedom for the rest of my days.
My sorrows, my disappointment, my expectations all banished;
In the blink of an eye, like a puff of smoke, they vanish.
I am more than I am;

This I now know.
As I shatter illusion
And finally see where to go:
To the stars up above
To the oceans so wide
Into a chasm of peace
Never again to hide
From the joy that is mine,
A feeling so pure
Ready to begin again
So quiet and demure.
A spark; no, a pulse; no, a beat of a heart.
And so, as has been for eons,
A brand-new start: rebirth.

———

My Vancouver doctor, Debbie, arrived at the house very late the next night. Jon was panicked and needed her advice. One look at me was all it took for her to know I had to go to the hospital. This time, *C. difficile* was confirmed. I was dehydrated from the throwing up and diarrhea, so I was hooked up to an IV and given five bags of fluid, along with special antibiotics to treat the infection. Jacqueline was not permitted to come anywhere near me because of the possibility of infecting either her or her family. I was released from the hospital the next day and spent a week in bed, quietly recovering. I ended up remaining on antibiotics for three years. Each time I tried to go off them, I had a recurrence of *C. difficile*. I could not understand why my body could not seem to clear this infection. I worried that I would become immune to the antibiotics, and then what would I do if they stopped working?

MY TRIP TO Vancouver was not what I had hoped it would be. I returned to Montreal exhausted from the ordeal but no longer in pain. I had become as fragile as glass. I did not want to go anywhere or see anyone. I was fearful of an attack happening anywhere, at any time. I needed constant reassurance that I was not making this up. Was I becoming paranoid? Could I be a hypochondriac? What was happening to me made no sense.

Every time Rubin saw me, he would put his hands on my belly. It was getting to the point that by simply touching me, he could tell whether I was going to obstruct. One evening, he and his wife, Marsha, picked me up to go to a party. After saying hello and touching my stomach, he looked at me and said, "Oh, no!" He knew that I was going to have a problem, as my belly had become hard and distended. He asked me if I was sure that I really wanted to go to the party. I said yes, because I had refused so many things and I was tired of disappointing Jon. In truth, I was bored with myself. I promised Rubin that I would not eat or drink anything. It was not a problem, since I had absolutely no appetite and was terrified to have anything pass my lips.

One hour was all I could last. The discomfort became hard to bear. I left with Jon, who refused to let me go home alone. I lay writhing in pain, curled up into a ball. Jon rubbed my back until Rubin arrived, drugs in hand. Marsha is an incredible woman. She never complained. I would call their house sometimes at 3 a.m. I've interrupted dinners and other evening activities, but she never said a word. You have to be a pretty special person to be a doctor's wife, because believe me, I definitely interfered with their home life for the better part of five years. I am so grateful for their friendship.

Jonathan had to go out of town on business a few days later, and he did not want me staying home alone. I refused to have anyone at the house, and my sister-in-law Diane, who lived around the corner, reassured him that she would come over at any time of the night if I was in trouble. It was almost as if Jon had a premonition of what was coming. At 4 a.m., after throwing up and suffering terrible spasms for two hours, I was forced to call Diane. She was over in minutes. One look was all it took before she called Rubin. He rushed over and we went to the hospital. He was furious at me for waiting so long to call him. I think he was angry because he couldn't stand to see me suffer any longer. I could not understand how he could be angry with me. I tried hard to manage the pain on my own. What was I going to do, call him every time I was in pain? I had some sort of pain most of the time. I felt as though I was abusing his good nature and our friendship. These attacks were now happening every six to eight weeks. If this was going to be my life, I wondered, how long could I keep it up? How much more pain can a human body withstand before it simply stops? Why did the doctors feel that nothing could be done for me? Living this way was pure insanity.

Nietzsche once said, "He who has a why to live for can bear with almost any how." Very few people really understood the depths of my suffering. It was not my nature to talk to everyone about how miserable I was. In truth, I was sick of myself. Why would I want to share any more than I had to with anyone else? I needed to constantly remind myself of why I wanted to keep going. I had gotten to see my beautiful girls graduate, not only from high school but from college, and become women in their own right. I had passed my fiftieth birthday. All I had ever wanted was the pleasure of watching my family expand and to see what kind of people my grandchildren would become. Each time I conquered one goal, I created a new one.

I continued to work between the attacks and tried to simply live my life as best I could. My clients understood when I was forced to cancel a session with them. They saw my attempts to implement all that I was teaching them on a daily basis. As much as I had hoped I was supporting them, it was they who seemed to be supporting me. Each time I worked with someone, it reminded me how to live my life as best as I could and to be grateful for what I had. Work became my drug of choice. But my patience with myself was wearing thin. If someone asked how I was feeling, I would simply say that everything was fine. I began retreating and disappearing into myself. I had just enough energy to take care of my family and see my clients.

I felt sorry for my husband. "Poor guy, he must really love me," I thought. He tried everything he could to make life easy for me. It was hard for him to see his happy-go-lucky wife losing some of her zest for life. Jon always prided himself on traveling to new destinations, and we rarely visited the same place twice. That is, until now. Here he was, renting the same house for us in St. Maarten year after year for the Christmas holidays. The purpose was to ensure I felt comfortable with the knowledge that there were daily flights back home if we needed to return quickly. St. Maarten was closer than Vancouver, and our friends who had a home there set us up with access to good medical care, should we need it. It was important for me to have a place that felt like home. I could fill my fridge with the foods that were good for me and take rest when necessary.

For Christmas 2008, Rubin, Marsha, and some other friends arrived to stay for a week. I was so grateful to have my good friends and my doctor there. I had tried every laxative and enema I could think of, but by the time they arrived, I had not gone to the bathroom for more than three weeks. It was weird; I had no pain but did not feel well. I had very little appetite. I had become good at hiding discomfort, and no one other than Rubin and Jon knew that I was having difficulties. Rubin kept trying different things to get me going, but nothing worked. The day before they were supposed to go home, all hell broke loose.

My belly became rock hard and blew up. I looked as though I was six months pregnant. The pain medication Rubin had on hand did not do the trick, and we both knew that I was in trouble. It amazed me how much I had been able to cope with. I so wanted to be able to enjoy St. Maarten. I loved being there and had so many wonderful people to spend time with. Again, my body was the one in charge. It demanded attention.

Rubin insisted that Jon book tickets for us to fly home with him the following day. He said that we had run out of options and that I needed to be hospitalized as quickly as possible. Chaos ensued. Normally, we rented the house for five weeks. This was only the end of the second week. We were forced to pack up the entire house and give all the food away in case we did not return. Everyone sprang into action. Phone calls were made, tickets were purchased, and the house was packed up before we knew it. Everyone had a job to do, except me. I couldn't move.

I lay in bed just trying to breathe. "Not again," my soul wept. I couldn't keep doing this. Something had to change. I began to think about how it might feel to have my entire bowel removed and to be forced to wear a colostomy bag. At that moment, it felt plausible. If it gave me my life back, I was finally willing to consider it. If I didn't like the way my belly looked before, what I might have to face could be a hell of a lot worse. It didn't matter; this was no life. Vanity be damned, it was sanity I was after. My girlfriend Diane was a calming force. She spoke slowly and quietly in the car as she drove Jon, Rubin, and me to the airport, while I curled my body into a little ball and tried somehow to find relief. Someone got me a wheelchair at the airport, as it was impossible for me to walk. Somehow I got on the plane. The person who was supposed to sit next to me was able to move so that I could have some extra space. I normally dislike flying and find it hard to sit still. This trip was quite different.

I puked, I writhed, I took drugs, and I slept. I remembered a joke about all the different organs in the body deciding which was the most important. The punch line was the colon, who thought that it was the most important because if it ceased to function, then all of the other organs would soon be full of shit. Quite funny, and oh so true, I thought. I was present during the flight home, but not really conscious of time or space. I must have looked quite horrific, because I was instantly wheeled through customs without anyone even bothering to look at my passport. Rubin drove me right to the Jewish General Hospital while Jon went home to pick up the things I might need.

There were no open beds on the medical or surgical floors, so it seemed curious that I ended up in a private room on a palliative care floor, where the hospital treats those who are close to death. "Me and them," I thought. "Are we really so different?" Some part of me was definitely dying. It felt as though my spirit and my optimistic nature were oozing out of my pores along with the sweat from my pain.

The week in the hospital was a nightmare. My daughter Kassy had never seen me in such a state. I had nothing left to keep it together. I cried and screamed, holding nothing back. What she saw was raw reality, and it was far from pretty. I think that the experience traumatized her to this day. She was terrified to leave me. The doctor's voices were serious, almost angry: "Why have you waited so long? We need to take care of this now. Your system is not functioning. We need to be aggressive." What was wrong with me that I could have done this to myself? *Did* I do this to myself? I had tried everything, but nothing had worked. I needed a plan B. I vowed this was never going to happen again. I had finally reached my breaking point. Hallelujah! What the hell took me so long? I knew something had to change. Someone had to have answers. I was not going to stop looking until I had exhausted all the possibilities. For the moment, however, I needed to deal with the situation at hand. I needed to be unblocked.

(15)

PUSHED
TO THE LIMIT

AS THE DOCTORS held me down and shoved instruments into me, memories of having been raped at seventeen came flooding back. I thought I had dealt with the trauma and put the experience behind me over the many years that followed. But now I screamed in pain as they constrained me. The memories filled my mind. I was unable to move as they did what was needed to unblock me. Tubes in and tubes out. I felt invaded in every orifice. "Stop, it hurts," I heard myself cry. "Breathe," they said. "We need to do this." "Stop, get it out," I screamed. "Relax, it will soon be done," they replied. I am sure the doctors and nurses must have thought twice about putting me in a palliative care unit. It was supposed to be a quiet and serene environment, and the noises emanating from my room were anything but. They were vile and definitely not good for those patients who were dying. I felt as though I was being raped all over again. This time was worse; this was a required raping. As I was held down, I realized that there was nothing I could do or say to stop the process. During my stay in the hospital, I wanted no one to see me. I forbade visitors. Anyone who walked through my doors invaded my personal hell. I hated the side effects of the morphine but gave in, for it left me with a feeling of peaceful indifference. It let me shut down, retreat, and disappear.

The process of cleaning out my colon went on for days. I was completely voiceless by the time it was over. I had no more fight left in me. Finally, six days later, after another gallon of what I like to call cleaning fluid was put down my nose through a tube into my stomach, it was over.

It was around 11 p.m., and Kassy was still there with me. My poor child had hardly slept or eaten the entire time I was in the hospital. She needed to keep vigil over me, as much for her sake as for mine. As horrible as it was for her, she was drawn into the drama and could not leave until it was over. Talk about an inability to protect your own child. Never in my wildest imagination would I have thought that any of my children would have had to witness the pure hell I had just experienced. A veterinarian would never have put an animal through what I had just suffered. They would have had mercy and put it to sleep. Kassy had trouble sleeping long after I left the hospital.

I pressed the button to call the nurse to let her know that the treatment was finished and that the tubes could be removed. It took her too long to answer. Couldn't she understand that even one more minute was more than I could bear? My daughter implored me to be patient and wait, but I could not. I ripped the tubes out as Kassy gasped. It felt as though I was pulling out my entrails. The tube down to my stomach was so long that it seemed to go on forever. I do not know where I got the courage, but I knew that I was on a mission. Next, out came the IV; I had seen it done so many times, it was a no-brainer.

At last, I was done. My life force was returning, and I wanted out. When the nurse finally arrived, she was alarmed that her compliant patient (it is easy to be compliant when you've had the life force sucked out of you) had turned into a defiant one. I told her I was leaving. She convinced me to wait until morning. Suddenly, I was too tired to argue. Just before I fell into a deep, dreamless sleep, I pictured that flower in my driveway. Both of us had made it against incredible odds. Both of us had survived.

MY COLORECTAL SURGEON, Carol-Ann, and my family doctor, Rubin, were puzzled by my case and knew they needed help finding answers. Internal investigations revealed that my colon had nothing obstructing its function. Why then wasn't it working? They recommended that I go to the Mayo Clinic for another opinion. The Mayo Clinic specializes in treating difficult cases, and people are referred there from across North America. The mission statement is to provide hope along with the best possible medical treatment and expertise. The clinic is well known for its innovative treatments and integrated whole person care. I was eager to see whether its doctors might be able to offer some valuable insight into my case. Never again was I going to go through what I had just experienced. I was prepared to live on a liquid diet for the rest of my life if need be. I was prepared to have my colon removed. I was prepared to do anything. I just couldn't survive a repeat of this story.

As Jon was unavailable, my girlfriend Gloria offered to go with me. I was afraid to go by myself. The Mayo Clinic has three locations: Arizona, Florida, and Minnesota. We chose the clinic in Jacksonville, Florida. I had no idea whether one location was better than the other, so I just chose the clinic that could see me the fastest. After two days of testing, the doctors felt that I had something called pelvic floor dysfunction. There are certain muscles that are supposed to relax when we have a bowel movement; instead, the doctors believed that mine were contracting. They could not tell for sure that this was the problem, but they wanted to rule it out. Apparently, my history led them to this conclusion. I didn't believe them for a moment and was quite disappointed by the diagnosis. But I decided that I was willing to try whatever they suggested. After all, this clinic was one of the most respected institutions in North America.

I was put on a medicine typically given to people with spinal cord injuries, something to pull more liquid into the intestines and make the stools very soft and loose. The idea is to help the bowels flow more easily. I was also told to do specific daily enemas, which caused me a great deal of internal pain. I went to a special clinic back home to learn a form of behavior modification to relax those particular muscles that the doctors felt were too contracted. It was not the most pleasant experience, but I followed every recommendation the doctors made. I was going to give it my best shot.

After months of physiotherapy and the daily practice of the assigned exercises, the physiotherapists at the clinic in Montreal told me that to the best of their knowledge, I didn't actually have the disorder, and they recommended that I stop treatment. In my heart, I knew they were right. I was back to square one, feeling more frustrated than ever. I needed a break from my life. I wanted to run away. The only problem was that I had to bring myself with me! There did not seem to be an end in sight. Two kinds of cancer hadn't killed me, but I wondered if these obstructions would result in my ultimate demise. If the experts could not find out what was wrong with me, what was I going to do?

I had been working for years with Linda Berthiaume, a homeopathic physician. She had told me years earlier that she thought that my problem required a surgical intervention. Now she felt that she had really exhausted all possibilities on her end. Great, even Linda was giving up on me. What was I going to do? The difficulty was that if I was going to have surgery, what were they going to operate on? There was no consensus among my doctors. Maybe it was time to simply remove the entire colon. Anything had to be better than what I was living with. For me to thrive, I needed to be hopeful and optimistic about the future. Who, after all, wants to imagine living a nightmare they will never wake up from? I refused to believe that there was no hope for me. There had to be an answer out there somewhere. I just needed to figure out where.

For one full year, I spent an hour each morning in the bathroom doing various procedures that had been recommended by my family doctor to keep me from getting blocked up. Until a solution could be found, he also thought that I should continue taking the medication that the Mayo Clinic had given me to keep my stools very soft. It was getting to the point that anything inserted rectally caused me tremendous spasms and local pain. I hated my morning routine and cried throughout it, but I convinced myself that once this task was done, I would have the freedom to enjoy the day. As long as I kept myself virtually empty, the bowel obstructions remained relatively under control.

In hindsight, I cannot believe how many years I put up with not feeling well. I wasted at least five years of my life in anguish. I could never have stood by and let it go on so long had it been my husband or kids who were suffering. If it were one of my clients, I would have advised them not to give up and to hunt for solutions as long as they were alive. Why did it take me so long to reach my breaking point? What was wrong with me? The situation was not rectifying itself, and I needed an intervention. One way or the other, I was determined to do whatever needed to be done to fix it. There was no turning back. If it meant the removal of my colon, then so be it. I was finally prepared. In cancer treatment, there are specific protocols to be followed depending on the type of cancer (chemotherapy, hormone therapy, or targeted therapies, for example). It is up to each individual to decide whether to follow them. This was a different story. No one had any answers. No one even had any more suggestions. Everyone was grasping at straws. On paper, my case simply did not make sense. Colonoscopies showed that everything was clear. Why then was my system not working?

Finally, I demanded a meeting with all the specialists who were independently working on me. At the beginning of November 2009, we gathered a team of doctors to create an action plan. There we were: Rubin, my family doctor; Carol-Ann, my colorectal surgeon; Hartley Stern, the director general of our hospital, whose clinical focus is colorectal cancer; a radiologist I had never met before; Mark Miller, a doctor from the infectious disease department (since I was still taking medication for *C. difficile*); and my husband and me. I told them I was done. I could not live like this any longer. It was beginning to eat at my soul. I had always been a happy and contented person, but I was losing that part of me. I was disappearing and becoming a recluse. Everyone agreed that something had to be done. The idea of a temporary colostomy (when a piece of healthy large intestine is attached outside the body on the abdominal wall and the feces empty into an external pouch) was finally put on the table. It was in the hope that I would have some relief from the pain and blockages while a permanent solution could be devised.

God bless Carol-Ann. This tiny woman, all of about five-foot-two, maybe weighing ninety pounds soaking wet, emphatically said no. She claimed that it would be difficult enough to cut into me once (with all the scar tissue she suspected to find), let alone twice. She needed to know exactly where the problem was before she would operate on me. She insisted that I see another doctor, Michael Camilleri, at the Mayo Clinic in Rochester, Minnesota. He was the world expert in the field and had mentored the doctor I had seen in Jacksonville, Florida. Carol-Ann had recommended I see him before, but it took so long to get an appointment that I went to see his colleague in Jacksonville instead.

At last, we had consensus. I wondered if everyone agreed because no one had anything else to suggest. It did not really matter. Appointments were made, and Jonathan and I planned to see the doctor in January 2010. I was so excited, I could barely wait.

It is hard to believe that I could still be hopeful after everything I had gone through, but I was. I'm not sure where the fire comes from, but for me, as long as possibility exists, that flame burns so brightly. It becomes my beacon of hope, lighting the way and propelling me forward. Thoughts of God automatically filled my mind. Was this a sign from him, I wondered? I felt the shackles of constriction start to break apart. Once again, I was reminded of that flower breaking though the asphalt in my driveway. I could sense its determination infusing each and every cell within my body. I felt strong, powerful, and alive. I felt myself breathe more fully. Perhaps that's what freedom is—the ability to start anew and be limitless in our thinking. All I know for sure is that as long as I am able to continue to believe that anything is possible, I can weather any situation.

———

· *patients' rights* ·

I WAS SO lucky to have a team of doctors ready to get together and try to figure out what to do with my case. I had a leader, my family doctor, who was able to coordinate the entire team. I wonder about all the patients who are frightened and scared, many of whom do not have an advocate championing their cause. Where can they go and who can they turn to for help with all the complex issues that accompany illness? Not everyone has the financial resources or the personal contacts I was lucky to have. In truth, had my doctors not been willing to come together and meet with me, I would have called the hospital ombudsman and registered a complaint, and she would have made the meeting happen. Each one of us, irrespective of who we know or what financial circumstances we face, has the right to get our needs met.

Patients need someone to speak up for them if they cannot speak for themselves. We need to encourage them to find every resource available to guide them through this process. And we need to enlist the aid of others to help us coordinate care. Social workers, hospital users' committees (patient advocacy groups for all those who use the hospitals), psychologists, librarians, and support groups can often help navigate through the maze of information that exists today. Patient advocacy groups play a vital role in guiding someone who is unwell. They are usually filled with people who themselves have been ill and offer the kind of resources and support that only someone who has really been there can offer.

It is too easy for a compliant patient to get lost in the system. We need to encourage one another to find our voices so that we may speak up without fear of reprisal. We must realize that our doctors are our partners, and their job is to help us as best they can. In order for them to do their job well, we also have to do our part. Medicine is sometimes limited in its resources. Society, however, is filled with many organizations that can help us. It is our job to find and use them.

———

MY LAST BOWEL obstruction occurred in November 2009. It was only ten days before the Angel Ball to celebrate the Jewish General Hospital's seventy-fifth anniversary, where I was to be honored for the work I had done with cancer patients. I wondered if I would even make it to my own event. Thank goodness I did, because this was very important to me. I have never loved being in the limelight and have always quietly done my work to the best of my ability. Everything I do, from private practice to hospital work to volunteering, I do because I love it, and I have never felt comfortable with a lot of praise. This time was different. I accepted the honor with the knowledge that a large sum of money raised from the evening would be allocated to a research program of my choice. I was thrilled, as this program could potentially help so many people who were dealing with cancer. I looked upon this event as my way of saying thank you for all the support I had received along the way. I was one of the lucky ones who survived, and I vowed to continue teaching and working with those who were suffering.

The evening was a success, and I was overjoyed that so many of the doctors I worked with attended. I never could have made it without their support. Well over a million dollars was raised that night. I chose to donate the money I was allocated to the

Rehabilitation Exercise Oncology Program (REOP). The REOP team is composed of physiotherapists and exercise physiologists. They not only offer hope to cancer patients but also help improve their lives by getting them moving and making then stronger. They do so by individually assessing each patient and creating unique programs of exercise depending on individual capacity and tolerance. Mary-Ann Dalzell is the clinical director of the program and is an expert in her field. The CURE Foundation (started by Diane Guerrera, a breast cancer survivor) matched my contribution, and REOP was launched. It is a collaboration between Hope & Cope and the Segal Cancer Centre at the Jewish General Hospital. Although REOP is a relatively new program, it appears to be well on its way to success.

Jon and I rented the house in St. Maarten for Christmas 2009. This time, it didn't bother me that I had to fill a suitcase with more than fifty disposable enema bags and other paraphernalia. For the first time since this journey with bowel obstructions began in 1994, I felt deep down inside that my ordeal would soon be over. I felt joyful. We now had a plan. The holidays were great and passed without incident.

Around the middle of January 2010, Jon and I went to the Mayo Clinic in Rochester to meet with Dr. Camilleri. Upon arriving at the clinic, we were greeted by a team. Some of my reports had been sent in advance, and we arrived armed with X-rays and a file filled with my medical history. Within minutes of examining me, Dr. Camilleri told me that I did not have pelvic floor dysfunction. He unquestionably disagreed with his colleague in Florida. Yeah! I knew it all along. I wasn't crazy. He said that by looking at the X-rays, he could tell there was a serious problem, and it didn't matter what I ate or didn't eat. This was beyond my ability to fix. Another yeah! This wasn't my fault. I got confirmation from the expert—and, of course, since it was in alignment with my beliefs, I liked what he had to say.

I felt so relieved. Illness is difficult enough without playing the blame game. It is disheartening to have everyone around you feel frustrated because they don't think that you are doing what you need to do to get better. You start doubting yourself, and that puts you in an even more vulnerable position. It did not matter how many times Rubin said it wasn't all in my head. Although I knew I was being irrational, I felt that I was partly responsible for my insides not working. It made me wonder how cancer patients must feel when their families don't think they are trying hard enough to get better. Illness is tough to deal with on its own, but the guilt created by the feeling that somehow you are not doing your best can truly be damaging to your spirit.

I stayed at the Mayo Clinic for a week. Some of the tests were extremely painful. I had already received the news that my small intestine was healthy, and even if the doctor had to remove the colon, he could attach the small intestine to the rectum and I would not need a colostomy bag. I was flying high. My father-in-law had worn a colostomy bag for six months while he was healing from a serious case of diverticulitis, a digestive disease in which there is a weakness in the lining of the colon that creates little pouches that can get inflamed or infected when they get blocked with waste products. In very serious cases, the pouches perforate, allowing waste products to spill into the abdominal cavity, potentially resulting in sepsis. He could barely look at himself in the mirror and was disgusted by the whole process. Although no one desires to have their colon removed, for some of my clients a colostomy bag simply becomes a means to an end, and for those in pain it is a blessed relief. Although I was willing to have the procedure if necessary, I wondered how I would handle it. We never know for sure what our reaction will be until we are actually faced with a situation. As much as I knew it could relieve many of my problems, I was glad that I would not have to face that reality.

It was time for the big test at the clinic, which was intended to check two things. The first was to see whether my brain was sending the proper message to the colon to create peristalsis (a necessary process of contractions that gently pushes the food through the digestive system). The second was to determine whether the nerves in my colon were healthy enough to receive the messages sent to them by the brain. In order to complete the test, it was essential to clean the bowel. The process was an exhausting and excruciating ordeal; the doctor had so much trouble cleaning me out that after a few hours, he told me with tears in his eyes that we both needed a break. It was only because I was from out of town that he even attempted to continue. He knew I was scheduled to go home the next day. He told me how sorry he was so for causing me so much pain. For this particular test, I was not allowed any pain medication as it would interfere with the impulses from the brain they were trying to test. I was not allowed to move and had to have three nurses hold me in place. The remnants of the ordeal were an exhausted team and a pool of sweat and tears around the table. The test took seven hours, and the doctor asked us to meet in his office an hour post-exam. The great thing about the Mayo Clinic is that if your test results are available, you get them immediately. I quickly cleaned myself up. After so many years of waiting, I was as excited as a child going for ice cream. "Finally," I thought, "maybe this can be fixed."

As we walked into Dr. Camilleri's office, he smiled and said, "Good news, we found it!" After carefully reviewing the data, the doctor determined that I had what is called a functional obstruction in the colon. It was difficult to figure out because the colon looked healthy and appeared to be open and functioning. Thanks to sophisticated technology, he was able to discover what area was not working properly. He said it was no wonder I couldn't get rid of the *C. difficile*; I was never cleaned out completely. There must have been bacteria festering in my colon for years. The solution was a surgical one, and it was quite simple. Just remove the affected area, sew the two parts together, and take the time to heal. I was beyond elated. As much as I hated the idea of being cut open again, I was looking forward to this operation.

Our plane was leaving the next morning, but Jon and I couldn't wait until we got home to make the arrangements for surgery. Carol-Ann and Rubin were waiting for our phone call and were so happy that we would finally be putting an end to this horrendous ordeal. Surgery was scheduled for three weeks later. That joyful part of me, which was so essential to keeping me alive, was awakening once again. That flower and I were not so different after all. We both just wanted to live. I felt my insides smiling. All of the hairs on my arms rose as if to give me a standing ovation. We had come such a long way and finally had an answer. In spite of it all, I hadn't given up. It may have taken me years longer than I would have liked, but here I was, finally, answer in hand. I was overcome with gratitude, and although my dad had died years earlier, I felt his arms wrapped tightly around me.

Our hotel was close to the Mall of America, a megamall that Jon wanted to see. Although I was exhausted, there was no way I would say no to him, especially after everything we'd been through. It was only while walking around with my husband that I let myself actually feel all that had transpired that week. I'd gone through hell but come out stronger on the other side. Hope resurfaced and infused every cell of my being. I had a chance to feel well again. Perhaps there might come a day when I wouldn't have that uncomfortable feeling of fullness in my belly. Although it was not always painful, it was always present. I walked serenely around this huge mall. Jon shopped until he dropped, so grateful to have good news for a change. I happily sat outside each store, calmly quiet and pensive, even though I was completely exhausted and shopping was the last thing on my mind. We ate a light dinner and went to bed early. I slept peacefully for the first time in a week.

(16)

RELIEF

THE SURGERY WAS scheduled for February 2010, around the same time as the Winter Olympics in Vancouver. Jon and I had been invited as VIP guests of a major Canadian corporation, and we had been very excited by the prospect of attending all the final events and closing ceremony. This was an opportunity that did not come around very often. Jon looked at me imploringly and asked whether I could postpone the operation for ten days so that we could go. I'm sure he felt that waiting ten days longer, after so many years, was not a lot to ask.

I just couldn't do it, and a part of me felt sorry for saying no. Although I appreciated how much he had sacrificed and accommodated me over the years, it was hard for me to understand how he couldn't see that once a solution was at hand, ten more days would have been too much for me to handle. I realized that as much as Jon had partnered me through all my ups and downs, I rarely talked to him about my deepest feelings and fears. I had been so private and stoic that I rarely shared with him the depths of my anguish. I am not sure that I even had the capacity to verbalize all that I felt, for even admitting it to myself was painful, let alone sharing it with anyone else.

Perhaps I thought he would not understand. Perhaps I wanted to protect him and myself from saying the words out loud. I am not sure.

All I knew was that I had been waiting more than fifteen years. It was only when I opened myself up to Jon that we both realized I had been holding on by just a thread. Our psyches can handle only so much, and I feared that any deviation from the plan would crack mine right open. It took everything inside me to wait the three weeks. Once I started being completely transparent, I think Jon finally understood the depths of my suffering. He never said another word about it. We would watch the Olympics together at home on television. They really were the best seats in the house, after all.

Preparation for surgery was difficult. Patients usually arrive at the hospital the morning of surgery or the night before. I was admitted two full days in advance. Two gallons of that familiar cleaning fluid went down a nasogastric tube over the two-day period. This time, I took it easily. I was hopeful and excited. Finally, everything was set. I had a team of caregivers ready to help me through the next ten days. I was good to go.

I asked my surgeon, Carol-Ann, whether she could fix the scars on my belly, or at least try to make them look a little bit better. I think she thought I was a bit of a looney tune, but hey, once I was being opened up, why not go for it? Unfortunately, she could not do what I would have liked. The operation turned out to be more complicated than a simple cut and re-stitch. The surgery lasted almost seven hours, twice as long as expected. Carol-Ann and her resident worked tirelessly, trying to get rid of as much scar tissue as they could. She had to cancel her next surgery because she was exhausted. Apparently, I was a real mess inside. Carol-Ann was right when she said that she did not want to go inside that belly of mine unless she absolutely had to. The amount of scar tissue she had to deal with was extensive.

Jon and Ali spent the entire day together waiting in the hospital. I was in the recovery room for a very long time before my family could see me. They were in agony, waiting, praying that nothing had gone wrong. I had an epidural block to ensure that I had no pain from the surgical site, but when I awoke my right arm was throbbing. I must have been lying in an awkward position during the surgery. All I could think of was my arm.

A friend of mine had had a team of caregivers stay with his mom during the last ten years of her life. They took care of her as though she was family. These are the women I had stay with me during my recovery, and I was very grateful to have them there to help me. Shelly Blackwood was a caregiving professional who put together a team of kind and loving women. They tended to my every need and made my family feel that I was safe and well looked after when they were not there.

Jon had been so worried (he feared that I was in serious trouble, because the operation had taken so long) and was so exhausted that, the day after surgery, he developed a terrible flu. He felt guilty about not visiting me for three days. I laughed, thinking that he needed the rest as much as I did. He had been keeping it together for all of us for a very long time. This was an opportunity for him to finally let go and spend some quiet time alone. He got a lot more than he bargained for when he married me, and now he too needed time to recover from all that had passed.

The first few days were very challenging. My blood pressure was extremely low, and the doctors pumped almost twenty pounds of fluid into me to raise it. Most patients are out of bed by the day after surgery. It took three days before I could leave my bed.

Alexandra was my only daughter living in Montreal at the time. Jacqueline was in Vancouver, and Kassy was attending acupuncture school in Florida. They asked if I needed or wanted them to come home, but I turned them down. I had everything in order and did not want anyone hovering. Ali had a young child to take care of and was very respectful of my space. I was grateful for her vigilance, as well as her distance. If I needed something, I knew I could count on her. She is so easy to be with. It was lovely getting to spend some quiet time just being close to her. She was the one I felt I knew the least when she was a young girl, since I was unable to devote as much time to her as I had to her sisters. She is smart and clearheaded. There is a part of her that reminds me so much of Jon. As for everyone else, I was happy to have very few visitors. I needed quiet and time to heal. I was not just healing from an operation; I was finally healing from more than thirty years of pain of one sort or another.

About five days after surgery, the magic happened. I went to the bathroom. Eureka!

I understand that for those who have never experienced a problem in this department, this is no big deal. For me, it was monumental. I could not hold back the tears. I got on the phone and called everyone I could think of to share the news. I could barely speak through the tears to get the news out. I wanted to announce to the world that I, Susan Wener, had had an effortless bowel movement! I was beyond joyful; I was euphoric. Even now, not a day goes by when I don't flush that toilet excited to see what I left behind.

And then I was allowed to start eating. After ten days of no food, I was fantasizing about everything I saw on television.

I even had a dream about eating a Big Mac, which was funny because I hadn't been to McDonald's in at least twenty years. And then breakfast arrived: one ounce of cottage cheese. Whoever was in the room at that time must have thought that I had lost a lot more than some body parts. It took me almost one hour to eat "the best cottage cheese of my life." It was funny, though, because the next day, cottage cheese didn't appeal to me at all. My taste buds were all screwed up. One minute something tasted good, and the next it tasted terrible. I wondered if it was related to all the pain medication I had been given. But none of that really mattered, because I was going to the bathroom. I was healing like a champ and knew that it was simply a matter of time for me to get back to myself. I had depleted my resources for years, and for the first time, I was not in a rush.

FINALLY, IT WAS time to go home. I couldn't wait. There I was, back in my safe place with my housekeeper, Beth, by my side. She was so good to me. We love each other and count on one another like family. I remember how scared she was in 1999, when she told me that she was pregnant. She had been working for me only a short while and must have feared that I would fire her. I sat her down and asked her if she wanted the baby. When she said yes, I made her promise that she would bring the baby to work with her every day for at least a year. It was a gift I will always cherish, to have had the joy a baby brings into the house. I love Beth's daughter, Nicole, and her big brother, Jonathan. I feel privileged to still be so close to all of them. Beth is an amazing woman with a huge, open heart. She is always ready to help in any way she can.

She knew that I loved my coffee in the morning, but no matter how many times she made it for me, I could not stand the taste. My taste buds were off, and I knew that I just needed to go slowly and all would heal in time. Just like a Jewish mother, Beth wanted to fatten me up. Every day, she attempted to seduce me into eating. She would spend hours in the kitchen preparing soups, vegetables, and fish she hoped I would like. Jon was pleased as punch, for he had a variety of choices when he came home from work each evening.

It took about a month for me to heal and regain my appetite. My physical body had been through a lot, but my emotional one was just beginning to learn to walk again. Until I wrote this story, I didn't realize the magnitude of how much I had suffered, both physically and psychologically. Again, the prediction of the palm reader came to my mind. At the age of twenty-seven, even the strongest of heart would have wondered whether they could meet the challenge of a future like this. Now, more than thirty years later, having lived what seemed an impossible feat, I am humbled by the potential of the human spirit. It is not just the physical body that carries us through. There is something sacred and intangible that exists within each of us. It is this something that pushes and propels the physical body forward. What is it that creates resiliency? What is it that keeps us going through the darkest of darks? Some call it faith, but I call it hope.

(17)

FREEDOM

IT WAS FEBRUARY 12, 2011, one year after the big surgery. Life felt freer for me than it had in many years. My bowels were functioning properly, and it had been fifteen months since my last bowel obstruction. My energy had returned and my weight was normal. I felt healthy, strong, and well. I was seeing an osteopath regularly to help me keep the scar tissue from coming back in my abdominal area. My work was thriving, my family growing. Jacqueline had two children and was pregnant with her third. Ali had one and was pregnant with her second. Kassy was in love with Martin, who had a beautiful son, and plans were being made for their wedding. I found myself enjoying life thoroughly. I was able to become the kind of grandmother I had always wanted to be and was tickled pink when my grandchildren squealed with delight whenever they saw me. I felt peaceful and fulfilled.

I was in Vancouver for Jonah's fifth birthday. Because I had spent so much time in Vancouver over the years, I had developed a network of friends there. I was having lunch with one of my newer ones one day, a young woman named Anna. She and my husband serve as trustees for a Canadian think tank called the Fraser Institute. We connected immediately at a conference and have remained friends since. We started talking about some of my hospital work, and she asked me if I wanted to visit a small private surgical center she was running. I jumped at the chance. The center seemed so well run and efficient. I met many of the doctors who worked there part time. There were also a few who chose to opt out of the government medical system and work there full time.

Anna introduced me to a wonderful plastic surgeon she had great respect for. He seemed kind and gentle and spent a lot of time doing pro bono work in poor countries. Jokingly, I lifted my shirt, showed him the scars on my belly, and said, "Can you fix this?" He sat down with me and spent the next thirty minutes telling me what he thought he could do. After all I had been through, it was hard to believe I was considering a scar revision. Was I so shallow that even after I'd finally got my life back, I still could not accept the way I looked? Was I tempting fate, as an osteopath had once told me?

When I called my husband, who was in Toronto, I burst into tears on the telephone. I could barely get the words out. Was it possible that I might be able to look at myself naked in the mirror and not have my past written across my belly? We talked for a long time. He was soft with me. There was no judgment in his voice. He told me the surgery would be my Valentine's Day present. If it was important to me, he wanted me to just go ahead and do it. I booked the surgery for February 15, 2011. I would need to stay overnight in the hospital and remain in Vancouver for two weeks afterwards. I walked around for the next few days in a daze. Jon was having a small medical procedure performed in Toronto the day before mine. I questioned myself about whether it was good timing for me to do this. I knew, however, that if I didn't do it now, I would never do it at all. This was not a whim. It was something I had wanted to do for more than twenty-one years. I knew that I needed to call Carol-Ann and ask for her advice. What if she thought it was a bad idea? Although I did not want to be disappointed, I knew that in order not to second-guess myself, I had to make the call.

Carol-Ann told me that she'd never realized how much my scars truly bothered me. As a surgeon, she basically did her work and got in and got out as quickly as she could. She tried to sew up the tissue nicely, but none of us knows how we will heal, and I was left with what I considered to be a mess. I guess after everything Carol-Ann's seen, it looked like a pretty minor mess to her. She told me that if she had known how important it was to me, she would have encouraged me to fix it long before. She gave me her blessing, and I was thrilled that I was going into the surgery with peace of mind.

It was weird having surgery without Jon close by. Jackie was quite pregnant, and I could only ask so much of her. I was basically on my own. Jackie took me to the hospital the morning of the surgery, kissed me, and said she would see me later. I'd tried to call Jon the night before, to see how he was doing, but hadn't been able to connect with him. I managed to reach him minutes before my operation and felt peaceful that I had heard his voice. He had passed a bad night but was preparing to get on a plane and come home to Montreal. I knew that he would feel better once he was in his own bed.

The doctor came in to mark me just before surgery. He used a magic marker to draw all over my belly. He would operate within the area of his markings. I had always been shy, and now standing naked in front of a stranger made me want to faint. The look of shock on my face when he brought out his camera made him laugh wholeheartedly. He promised that my face would not appear in the pictures. He was not interested in my face, after all. It was the before-and-after pictures of my abdomen that he wanted.

The surgery was grueling. It stretched from one hour, to two, to more than three. I had so much scar tissue that he not only opened me up from hip to hip but lifted the skin, scraping off the scar tissue all the way up to my sternum. He told me afterwards that had he realized what the job would entail, he probably would not have agreed to do it. He made me a new belly button but told me that I would probably be left with some scars around where the old belly button was, because I was thin and there was no excess skin to get rid of.

It did not matter. I was so grateful to Anna for introducing me to this wonderful man. When he changed the bandages the next day, I was amazed. My belly was smooth and flat. My new belly button was beautiful. I told him that this was the first time in more than twenty-one years that I felt beautiful. I started to cry and was unable to stop for a long time. It had been a very painful operation, but I was not worried. I understood pain; it did not scare me. I knew that I would recover in time.

Jon, however, was not doing well. His operation had resulted in a tear in his diaphragm and caused him to bleed into the lining of his right lung. He was having a lot of trouble breathing, and his health was seriously compromised. He needed to be admitted to hospital days after he returned to Montreal. I knew that I needed to get home as quickly as I could. Although it was not ideal, I was given permission to travel one week after surgery.

Jon and I were quite the team. Although I had more than a hundred stitches inside and out, my issues seemed minor in comparison to his. I remembered what it was like to struggle for breath, and watching him now was difficult. I was grateful to be able to support him, for a change. He had been there for me so many times in the past. It was the least I could do now.

In time, both of us healed. I remember watching the Academy Awards with him and our friend Sal, saying that I had something in common with all the movie stars: plastic surgery seemed to be the common denominator. Jon laughed and said that the only difference was that nobody would ever see mine. That was the truth. I did not do it for anyone else. Jon never thought I needed it. To him, I was beautiful, with all my little flaws. This was just about me. I gave myself permission to fix what I did not like. It was a gift to me. It allowed me to physically let go of a landscape of the past that had caused me so much pain. Although I have some scarring from the surgery, it doesn't bother me at all. I feel beautiful.

SINCE I WAS feeling so well, Jon decided it was time to get on with our lives. He felt that we had put them on hold for a long time, and he was tired of traveling without me. He wanted to go away on a six-week adventure for Christmas 2011. It would be the first time in many years that I considered venturing far from home. I was terrified and tried everything I could to get him to change his mind. If I was really going to be free from my past, however, I couldn't just wet my toes; I had to jump into life with both feet. As scared as I was, part of me was ready. It was time not just to turn the page of an old story but to create a new one altogether.

In the past, I had refused to go anywhere that required shots of any kind. Now here I was, off to the tropical disease center to see what I needed to take to be safe in South America.

We were going to Brazil, Argentina, and Chile. The part I was most excited about was the jungle. I couldn't wait to learn all about the medicinal plants and hear all the stories from the guides who lived there. I wasn't just going away; I was going to the Amazon. Talk about a leap of faith!

I met with Linda, my homeopathic physician, and stocked up on all kinds of remedies. I think any bug or germ would have been scared to death to come within a hundred feet of me. I was armed to the hilt! My husband was not too impressed when we had to take another suitcase "just in case." I was prepared for anything. I had enough medication for a tribe, let alone one person.

I was scared until I got on the plane. As soon as it took off, however, I was at peace. I am not the most adventurous person by nature, and Jon has often had to push me to experience new things. Once I am there, though, I thrive and never look back. When the plane started its descent into the Amazon, I was mesmerized. We were above a tributary flowing into the Amazon. It looked black and muddy (that is why they call it the Rio Negro), whereas the Amazon itself was clear and bright. The Amazon and the Negro have different pH balances, and the animals that live in one would not survive in the other. The pink dolphins seem to be the exception. It is incredible to me that the separation is only that—a shift in pH—and everything living within each body of water is different. I am in awe of the magic of nature.

I had the vacation of a lifetime. I ate dinners much later than I was used to. I was able to skip, without consequences, the back stretches and special exercises that I'd had to do ever since having my spine fused. One night, we danced salsa at a local club until three in the morning. I felt at home in the jungle, sweating in hundred-degree weather with one hundred percent humidity. I saw more medicinal plants than I could name. I saw killer ants and bugs that I swear seemed as large as me, and I loved every single second of it all. I experienced a kind of freedom that I did not know was possible. I felt free from myself, from my own restrictions. I no longer needed to run away from myself. I laughed and giggled like a little girl. We just had so much fun!

When I look back over the years, I find it hard to believe how much I have grown. I would not have necessarily chosen illness as the vehicle to push me forward, but it was the one I got. In spite of it all, I have not only survived but thrived.

(18)

AFTERMATH

THE SUMMER OF 2012 was a joyous one. Kassy married a wonderful man who, along with his son, made an incredible addition to our family. In early December, they blessed us with a beautiful baby boy, raising our number of grandchildren to seven.

It is now September 2013. In March, I turned sixty years old. The thought of reaching that milestone never even entered my consciousness so many years ago. I am strong, healthy, and determined. I am thriving.

What will my future hold? I have no idea. What I do know is that I am excited to wake up each day. I look around and feel blessed. I have the most loving and supportive partner, whom I can't wait to cuddle up with at the end of the day. My children fill me with awe. They have become three of the most powerful, loving, and compassionate women I have ever met. The experiences they have gone through have given them wisdom that enables them to help so many people. Each of them, in her own way, makes the world a better place. My grandchildren fill me with wonder and allow me over and over again to see the world anew through their magical lenses. Their delight in life tickles my soul. Spending time with them is a gift I never take for granted. The rest of my family and friends are like soup for my soul. They warm my heart and are continuously nurturing and supportive.

And then there is you. You who are afraid. You who are suffering. You who are wondering what your fate might be. Pain and suffering are difficult. No one would willingly choose to experience them. Yet if we can simply surrender and step into the moments of our deepest anguish, we might be able to access a collective power greater than we ever thought possible. It is from this place of suffering that heroes emerge. We often hear stories of people finding incredible strength under the direst of circumstance. Surrendering is not about giving up. It's about experiencing life, with all its ups and downs. It is not about judging whether the situation is good or bad, fair or unfair. It is about finding moments of peace, even among all the mess. Pain and suffering are simply part of life, part of what make us who we are. No matter how hard we try, we will never be able to avoid them. Human beings were not meant to shed their skins over and over again like the snake does. But sometimes, the school of hard knocks forces us to do just that. It makes us break the shackles that keep us bound physically, mentally, and spiritually. It may help us move toward a place of freedom.

None of us can be certain what lies in store for us. What we do know is that even when the rug is pulled out from under our feet, we are capable of getting up. No system of medicine is perfect, and it is sometimes difficult to navigate through the myriad of choices that exist. We are able to learn from each one, however, taking only those aspects that resonate deeply inside us. Don't be afraid to explore. Don't be afraid to try, for it is through these efforts that doors open.

When people ask if I would do it over again, knowing what I would have to go through, I tell them I am not sure I would sign up. When people ask if it was worthwhile to have gone through it all to be where I am today, I smile. YES, it was worth it. True, I wish that I never had to deal with all that pain and suffering. I wish I could take back the distress those who love me had to endure. And I wish that this experience did not have to be the one that propelled me forward. But wishes don't always come packaged in the way we hope.

I am no longer an innocent young woman, but I am not jaded either. I carry my tool bag of strategies with me wherever I go. They remind me to keep one foot in front of the other. And I still believe, perhaps naively, that each day holds an opportunity for magic. I have grown so much from all that has passed. Today, when I look into the mirror, I like the woman I see reflected there. "You have come a long way, baby," I hear her say, no longer in spite of but because of it all.

And finally, if I can leave you with one last thought, it is this: Go out there and get your needs met. Remember that you are limitless in your potential. Be much more attached to the journey than the outcome. And don't be afraid to reach out and touch one another, for the gifts of kindness and compassion are far more contagious than any disease.

RECOMMENDED READING

Adair, Margo, and William Aal. *Practical Meditation for Busy Souls* (Naperville, IL: Sourcebooks, 2008).

Alexander, Eben. *Proof of Heaven: A Neurosurgeon's Journey into the Afterlife* (New York: Simon and Schuster, 2012).

Bach, Richard. *Jonathan Livingston Seagull* (New York: Scribner, 2006).

Bass, Ellen, and Laura Davis. *The Courage to Heal: A Guide for Women Survivors of Child Sexual Abuse* (New York: Harper Collins, 1988).

Benson, Herbert. *Timeless Healing: The Power and Biology of Belief* (New York: Scribner, 1997).

Benson, Herbert, and William Proctor. *The Relaxation Revolution: The Science and Genetics of Mind Body Healing* (New York: Scribner, 2011).

Chernin, Kim. *The Hungry Self* (New York: Harper Perennial, 1994).

Chopra, Deepak. *Perfect Health: The Complete Mind/Body Guide*, rev. ed. (New York: Harmony, 2001).

Cousins, Norman. *Anatomy of an Illness as Perceived by the Patient* (New York: W.W. Norton, 2005).

David, Marc. *Nourishing Wisdom: A Mind-Body Approach to Nutrition and Well-Being* (New York: Harmony, 1994).

Doidge, Norman. *The Brain That Changes Itself: Stories of Personal Triumph from the Frontiers of Brain Science* (New York: Penguin, 2007).

Dyer, Wayne. *You'll See It When You Believe It: The Way to Your Personal Transformation* (New York: Avon, 2001).

Ellis, George. *The Breath of Life: Mastering the Breathing Techniques of Pranayama and Qi Gong* (Career Books, 2000).

Fields, Rick. *Chop Wood, Carry Water: A Guide to Finding Spiritual Fulfillment in Everyday Life* (New York: Tarcher, 2002).

Gendlin, Eugene T. *Focusing* (New York: Bantam, 1987).

Gibran, Kahlil. *The Prophet* (New York: Knopf, 1923).

Hammer, Leon. *Red Bird Flies, Phoenix Rises: Psychology & Chinese Medicine* (Seattle: Eastland Press, 2005).

Harricharan, John. *When You Can Walk on Water, Take the Boat* (New York: Berkley Books, 2012).

Harris, Barbara, and Lionel C. Bascom. *Full Circle: The Near-Death Experience and Beyond* (New York: Pocket Books, 1993).

Hendricks, Gay. *The Art of Breathing and Centering: Discover the Powerful Gifts of the Air You Breathe* (New York: Macmillan, 2005).

Hicks, Esther, and Jerry Hicks. *The Astonishing Power of Emotions: Let Your Feelings Be Your Guide* (New York: Hay House, 2007).

Hirshberg, Caryle, and Marc Ian Barasch. *Remarkable Recoveries: What Extraordinary Healings Can Teach Us About Getting Well and Staying Well* (London: Headline, 1995).

Hoff, Benjamin. *The Tao of Pooh* (New York: Penguin, 1983).

Jahnke, Rodger. *The Healer Within: Using Traditional Chinese Techniques to Release Your Body's Own Medicine* (New York: HarperOne, 1998).

——. *The Healing Promise of Qi: Creating Extraordinary Wellness through Qigong and Tai Chi* (New York: McGraw-Hill, 2002).

Kabat-Zinn, Jon. *Full Catastrophe Living: Using the Wisdom of Your Body to Face Stress, Pain and Illness* (New York: Delta, 1990).

Kubler-Ross, Elisabeth. *On Death and Dying* (New York: Scribner, 1997).

——. *The Wheel of Life: A Memoir of Living and Dying* (New York: Scribner, 1998).

Moody, Raymond. *The Light Beyond* (New York: Bantam, 1989).

Rinpoche, Sogyal. *The Tibetan Book of Living and Dying* (New York: HarperOne, 1994).

——. *Glimpse after Glimpse* (New York: HarperOne, 1995).

Schatz, Hales Sofia, and Shira Shaiman. *If the Buddha Came to Dinner: How to Nourish Your Body to Awaken Your Spirit* (New York: Hyperion, 2004).

Smith, Manuel J. *When I Say No, I Feel Guilty* (New York: Bantam, 1985).

Spiegel, David. *Living Beyond Limits: New Hope and Help for Facing Life-Threatening Illness* (Boulder, CO: Bull Publishing, 2005).

Vanzant, Iyanla. *Peace from Broken Pieces: How to Get Through What You're Going Through* (New York: Smiley Books, 2012).

Vaughn, Frances. *Gifts from a Course in Miracles* (New York: Tarcher, 2002).

Walsch, Neale Donald. *Conversations with God: An Uncommon Dialogue* (New York: Putnam, 2002).

Mariechild, Diane. *The Inner Dance: A Guide to Spiritual and Psychological Unfolding* (Berkeley, CA: Crossing Press, 1987).

Merrett, Charles. *Relaxation Rules* (Mind's Eye Books, 1982).

Millman, Dan. *Way of the Peaceful Warrior: A Book That Changes Lives* (Tiburon, CA: HJ Kramer, 2006).

Ortzen, Tony. *The Seed of Truth*, Silver Birch Series (Oxhott, UK: Spiritual Truth Press, 1998).

——. *A Voice in the Wilderness*, Silver Birch Series (Oxhott, UK: Spiritual Truth Press, 2000).

Osborne, T.L. *Healing the Sick: A Living Classic* (Tulsa, OK: Harrison House, 1986).

Pelletier, Kenneth R. *Mind as Healer, Mind as Slayer* (New York: Delta, 1923).

Zukav, Gary. *Seat of the Soul* (New York: Free Press, 1990).

INDEX